Pediatric Voice

A Modern, Collaborative Approach to Care

Pediatric Voice

A Modern, Collaborative Approach to Care

Lisa N. Kelchner, PhD, CCC-SLP, BRS-S
Susan Baker Brehm, PhD, CCC-SLP
Barbara D. Weinrich, PhD, CCC-SLP

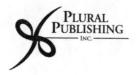

PLURAL
PUBLISHING
INC.

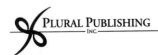

5521 Ruffin Road
San Diego, CA 92123

e-mail: info@pluralpublishing.com
Web site: http://www.pluralpublishing.com

Copyright © by Plural Publishing, Inc. 2014

Typeset in 11/13 Adobe Garamond by Achorn International
Printed in the United States of America by McNaughton & Gunn, Inc.

For permission to use material from this text, contact us by
Telephone: (866) 758-7251
Fax: (888) 758-7255
e-mail: permissions@pluralpublishing.com

Every attempt has been made to contact the copyright holders for material originally printed in another source. If any have been inadvertently overlooked, the publishers will gladly make the necessary arrangements at the first opportunity.

Library of Congress Cataloging-in-Publication Data

Kelchner, Lisa N., author.
    Pediatric voice : a modern, collaborative approach to care / Lisa N. Kelchner, Susan Baker Brehm, Barbara Weinrich.
        p. ; cm.
    Includes bibliographical references and index.
    ISBN-13: 978-1-59756-462-5 (alk. paper)
    ISBN-10: 1-59756-462-1 (alk. paper)
    I. Brehm, Susan Baker, author. II. Weinrich, Barbara Derickson, author. III. Title.
    [DNLM: 1. Voice Disorders—diagnosis. 2. Child. 3. Voice—physiology. 4. Voice Disorders—therapy. WV 500]
    RF510
    616.85'56—dc23
                                                                                  2013035348

Contents

Acknowledgments

We would like to thank our colleagues and friends, Stephanie Zacharias, PhD; Janet Beckmeyer, MA; and Janet Middendorf, MA, at the Center for Pediatric Voice Disorders, Cincinnati Children's Hospital Medical Center for their continuous support and collaboration during all our research and writing endeavors. We especially want to acknowledge Dr. Ann Kummer and Dr. Robin Cotton for providing us the opportunity to help create one of the most unique pediatric voice treatment programs in the country. As a team, we are committed to collaboratively serving our very special patient population to the best of our ability each and every day.

Four outstanding professionals made important contributions to the content of this book. Dr. Alessandro de Alarcon, Medical Director of the Center for Pediatric Voice Disorders, was the principal author of Chapter Four, Etiology and Management of Pediatric Voice Disorders. Dr. Wendy LeBorgne, Director of the Professional Voice Center of Greater Cincinnati and the Blaine Block Institute for Voice Analysis and Rehabilitation, Dayton, Ohio, authored the section on caring for the child and adolescent performer in Chapter Six. Special thanks to Keiko Ishikawa, MM, MA, accomplished doctoral student at the University of Cincinnati, for writing the section on vocal fold microstructure in Chapter Two and the Supplement on Wound Healing and the Vocal Folds. Aliza Cohen, Department of Pediatric Otolaryngology, Cincinnati Children's Hospital Medical Center, was an important mentor and editor. Her talents and contributions were invaluable.

The authors also want to acknowledge the contributions of three outstanding students, Melanie Reynolds and Annie Dillard (Department of Speech Pathology and Audiology at Miami University) and Emily Rayburn (Department of Communication Sciences and Disorders at the University of Cincinnati). Their tireless and capable reviews of the chapters kept reminding us of our most important audience, future clinicians.

Finally, and most importantly, to Todd, Jeff, Jen, Michael, Mom, Martin, Gregory, Tom, Zachary, Elizabeth, and Lan, thank you for your constant love, support, and understanding.

Lisa N. Kelchner, PhD, CCC-SLP, BRS-S
Susan Baker Brehm, PhD, CCC-SLP
Barbara D. Weinrich, PhD, CCC-SLP

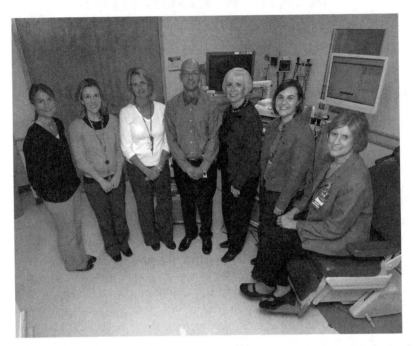

Center for Pediatric Voice Disorders Team at Cincinnati Children's Hospital Medical Center.

Contributors

Alessandro de Alarcon, MD, MPH
Director
Center for Pediatric Voice Disorders
Cincinnati Children's Hospital Medical Center
Associate Professor
Otolaryngology-Head and Neck Surgery
University of Cincinnati Department of Pediatrics
Cincinnati, Ohio
Chapter 4

Susan Baker Brehm, PhD, CCC-SLP
Associate Professor
Department Chair
Department of Speech Pathology and Audiology
Miami University
Oxford, Ohio

Keiko Ishikawa, MM, MA
Doctoral Student
University of Cincinnati
Cincinnati, Ohio
Chapter 2 and Appendix A

Lisa N. Kelchner, PhD, CCC-SLP, BRS-S
Associate Professor
Director of Graduate Studies
Department of Communication Sciences and Disorders
University of Cincinnati
Cincinnati, Ohio

Wendy D. LeBorgne, PhD, CCC-SLP
Voice Pathologist and Singing Voice Specialist
Adjunct Assistant Professor
Musical Theater
Cincinnati College-Conservatory of Music
University of Cincinnati
Cincinnati, Ohio
Clinical Director

The Blaine Block Institute for Voice Analysis and Rehabilitation
The Professional Voice Center of Greater Cincinnati
Dayton, Ohio
Chapter 6

Barbara Weinrich, PhD, CCC-SLP
Professor
Department of Speech Pathology and Audiology
Miami University
Oxford, Ohio

To all the children who begin life with special needs and challenges—
Let your voices be heard.

CHAPTER 1

Introduction

An infant's first cry is its announcement to the world that it has arrived. A loud, vibrant cry is the first indicator of a baby's health and well-being. Shaped by rapidly evolving skills, the voice of an infant conveys need, distress, and contentment. The future and integrity of that voice relies on an exquisite, highly timed, rapidly unfolding developmental process that works in coordination with neurologic, auditory, respiratory, and speech and language mechanisms. When an infant or child's development is interrupted or the mechanics of voice are altered, significant communication obstacles can occur. Understanding how the biologic, behavioral, and emotional functions of voice subserve communication and reflect health is an essential component of pediatric voice care.

A common phrase in pediatric medicine is that a child is not a miniature adult; that is, it is not enough to simply modify knowledge pertaining to adults and apply it to the care of children. Although the scientific underpinnings of voice production remain the same over the course of a lifespan, care of the pediatric voice requires knowledge of childhood developmental anatomy and physiology; growth and learning; educational, behavioral, parent, and family issues; and the potential for a voice disorder to have handicapping effects in classroom and social situations. More-over, taking care of the pediatric population entails specific approaches to evaluation and treatment.

Interestingly, most instructors of graduate courses in voice disorders use textbook(s) that provide the fundamentals of voice care and principles of voice science framed by cases and examples derived from the adult population; relatively little emphasis is placed on childhood voice disorders and care. Yet, many students will work in an early intervention or educational work setting. Once in such settings, these newly trained professionals may lack confidence in assessing and addressing pediatric voice problems. Furthermore, in the school setting, care of the child with a voice disorder may be considered a low priority or may not be considered a hindrance or educational handicap at all. In view of these issues, this book is designed to guide the reader through the development of a well-defined knowledge base that is essential to successful clinical practice in pediatric voice.

Throughout the text the reader will note a strong emphasis on a collaborative approach to the care of children with voice disorders. The authors of this book are fortunate to be able to care for their patients in an environment in which physicians and allied health professionals work hand in hand to provide well-integrated, comprehensive care. We have, however, kept in mind that many clinicians do not have that opportunity; this is reflected in some of the case-based examples we have presented.

This book follows a format that is similar to many traditional clinical disorder texts. The relevant anatomy and physiology, including the physiology of voice production, are reviewed in Chapter 2, followed by a discussion of pertinent neuroanatomy and physiology in Chapter 3. Chapter 4 covers all of the common (and some uncommon) etiologies associated with pediatric voice disorders and how they are medically and/or surgically managed. A comprehensive review of the pediatric voice evaluation is presented in Chapter 5, followed by a detailed discussion of treatment approaches in Chapter 6, which includes treatment and special considerations for the child performer as well. The final chapter is dedicated to the application and extension of information in the preceding chapters to the child who has a history of complex airway and voice disorders. Much of this chapter is dedicated to treatment and management considerations for children who were premature and were tracheotomized at one time. That is a population that will likely have a voice disorder that lasts a lifetime. Finally, an overview of wound healing is presented in an appendix at the end of the book. This section provides important information about the critical components of vocal fold injury and the process of tissue recovery at the cellular level.

The actual patient samples and examples we have provided are designed to offer some experience, in the sense that the reader will have the opportunity to do both auditory-perceptual and video-imaging ratings. We hope that listening and in some cases rating the samples will provide spe-cific insights and suggestions for the graduate student, as well as the school-based and solo practitioner. Each chapter contains an in-depth discussion of the fundamentals required to provide appropriate, high-quality care. *Why* a specific treatment approach is decided upon is as important, if not more so, as *how* a management plan is carried out. Although technical skills develop with experience, failure to understand the rationale of a treatment approach or technique will limit a clinician's ability to provide the best possible care. Providing optimal care almost always involves blending evidence supported, time-tested approaches with new trends. We have included updates on the ever-changing technology used in assessment and treatment, as well as novel models of voice care delivery, such as gaming and telehealth options. At the end of Chapters 5 (evaluation), 6 (treatment), and 7 (complex voice and airway patients), the reader will find case study examples that build upon knowledge presented in the text. The reader will also find "clinical notes" throughout some chapters that highlight important clinical concepts and extend knowledge in specific areas. In some chapters the reader will find references to the accompanying DVD that provides opportunities for practice of audio-perceptual ratings and stroboscopy ratings. Additional written, video, and audio examples of specific evaluation and therapy techniques are included on the DVD as well.

In conclusion, the purpose of this textbook is to provide practical information that is applicable to the clinician providing pediatric voice care. It is our hope that the insights gained will facilitate improved, comprehensive care of children with voice disorders in both early childhood and school-age educational settings.

CHAPTER 2

Anatomy and Physiology of the Pediatric Upper Aerodigestive Tract, Larynx, and Respiratory System

The laryngeal airway has three primary biologically related functions: (1) serving as a conduit for airflow during ventilation; (2) valving or sealing (and thus separating the upper from the lower respiratory tract) for airway protection or to increase subglottic pressure for straining and lifting; and (3) generating sound for phonation. Understanding the hierarchy of these functions is essential, as the order of their importance can determine needed interventions. For example, establishing a patent or adequate airway in a child is essential to survival and thus will be managed over voicing needs. This issue is revisited several times throughout this book as medical-surgical interventions and outcomes are presented.

This chapter provides the necessary fundamental information related to the anatomy and physiology of voice in the developing child. A child is not a miniature adult; therefore, an understanding of the rapid changes involving the structures and functions of the laryngeal and respiratory systems across childhood is required. A discussion of the anatomy and physiology of the head and neck is presented including the primary skeletal structures or framework (bones and cartilage), spaces, muscles, blood supply, nerves (innervation), and mucosal membranes. Of note, because the anatomy and the physiology of the oral cavity, tongue, and face are covered in basic anatomy courses that information is not repeated here. This section includes information about typical embryologic and postnatal development of the upper aerodigestive tract and lower respiratory tract structures, laryngeal histology, and the physiology of phonation. Specific information about the neural controls is covered in Chapter 3.

Anatomy of the Upper Respiratory System: Overview of Embryologic Development

To best understand the structures and what they do, it is important to first review their embryology. The transformation of the human embryo to newborn requires an elaborate, complicated, and exquisite biologic series of highly timed events. The respiratory system appears at approximately 3 weeks postconception (Larsen, 1993) following the differentiation of the embryo's rostral (toward the head) and caudal (away from the head) ends and the earliest development of the neural tube. The appearance of the pharyngeal arches (Figure 2–1) occurs at 4 weeks and will ultimately become the structures of the pharynx and the larynx. There are six pharyngeal arches; however, the fifth is considered rudimentary (Moore, 1992).

Pharyngeal arches are also referred to as branchial arches, a term that links embryologic development to primitive evolutionary processes. For every (outer) pharyngeal arch there is a corresponding (inner) pharyngeal pouch. Between the pharyngeal arch/pouch is a pharyngeal cleft. Each arch has a central core of mesenchyme or mesoderm, which is the cellular (or germ) layer between the endoderm (innermost germ layer) and ectoderm (outermost germ layer). Mesoderm gives rise

to connective tissue, muscles, bone, and circulatory and urogenital systems. Ectoderm gives rise to the epidermis (skin) and epidermal tissue, including the nervous system, glands, and mucous membranes of the mouth. Endoderm gives rise to the epithelial linings of the respiratory and digestive tracts as well as internal organs (e.g., liver and pancreas) and some glands.

The cartilaginous and bony structures of the face, mandible, larynx, and trachea arise from the mesoderm of the first, second, third, fourth, and sixth pharyngeal arches. The corresponding ectoderm gives rise to the cranial nerves, and the endoderm gives rise to respiratory and digestive tract organs as well as certain glands (Table 2–1).

The embryo to fetal transformation begins at week 8 and by that time the differentiation of the laryngeal cartilage and muscles is well under way (Bluestone et al., 2003; Larsen, 1993). Morphologically, all of the structures of the larynx, trachea, and digestive tract are present by (fetal) week 12 or the end of the first trimester. At this point, all of the structures are in their relative postnatal positions, although not fully developed, and the larynx and pharynx should now be a continuous recanalized tube. In months 3 through 6, intrauterine growth of the pharynx and trachea and midline fusion of the larynx occur along with differentiation and maturation of the muscles, nerves, and glandular structures. By the seventh month, the upper aerodigestive tract, including the laryngeal apparatus, is prepared to perform necessary biologic functions of life (Bluestone et al., 2003).

Observations of physiologic activity involving the head and neck have been observed via ultrasound technology. Between the ages of 9 and 12 weeks, the fetus is observed to swallow (amniotic fluid), produce suckle motions, and demonstrate respiratory movement of the pharynx, larynx, and diaphragm. After 13 weeks, activities such as lip opening, finger

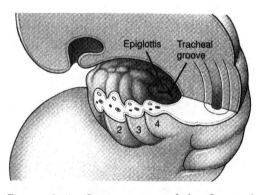

Figure 2–1. Cutaway view of the floor of the embryonic pharynx at approximately 4 weeks, showing pharyngeal arches 1 through 4, the laryngotracheal groove, and the origin of the epiglottis. From Myer, Cotton, & Schott, 1995. Reprinted with permission from Lippincott, Williams & Wilkins.

Table 2–1. Developmental Overview of Early Embryologic Development of the Pharyngeal Arches and Grooves

Arch/Pouch	Endoderm	Mesoderm	Ectoderm/Arch
1st	Epithelial lining of the oral cavity, glands of anterior oral cavity	Bones of the upper and lower jaw MM mastication	CN V, trigeminal
2nd	Palatine tonsils, thyroid gland	Upper portion of hyoid bone MM facial expression Tongue	CN VII, facial
3rd	Epithelial lining of the pharynx, thymus gland	Contributes to hyoid Stylopharyngeus	CN IX, glossopharyngeal
4th	Lining of the hypopharynx, esophagus	Laryngeal cartilages Pharyngeal constrictors, levetor vili palatine	CN X, vagus (superior laryngeal)
6th	Lining of the larynx, trachea, esophagus	Laryngeal cartilages Intrinsic laryngeal MM Striated MM of the upper esophagus	CN X, vagus (recurrent laryngeal)

Legend: MM or mm = muscle.

suckling, and face touching can be observed (Miller, 2003). Failures of the embryologic and fetal developmental process at any time can result in structural and mechanical deficits that will be present at birth or observed during fetal development via ultrasound. Given its multiple essential functions, the aerodigestive region is vulnerable to intrauterine developmental failures caused by environmental or congenital factors.

Clinical Note: Failure of the larynx to recanalize, or open as a tube, can present as congenital laryngeal or subglottic stenosis, laryngeal web, or, if it fails to fuse at midline, a laryngeal cleft. If there is restriction of the laryngeal airway, a newborn infant will have difficulty breathing and a distinctly different cry (e.g., high pitched, weak). In the case of a deep laryngeal cleft, there may be problems with airway protection during feeding, as liquid can enter the posterior larynx below the level of the true vocal folds (TVFs).

Anatomy of the Upper Aerodigestive Tract: Overview of Postnatal Anatomy and Developmental Changes

At birth, the anatomy of the infant's head and neck include the same "parts" as that of an older child and adult, but they are proportioned differently and are not yet controlled by sophisticated, established sensory motor pathways. The infant skull is softer and not completely fused, and the position of the mandible is relatively level with the skull base (Meyer, Cotton, & Shott, 1995). The oral cavity is smaller and the tongue fills much of the oral cavity space. The pharynx is short and the position of the larynx within this region is relatively high and approximates cervical spine levels C1–C4. The epiglottis is upright with its tip able to touch and interlock with the velum during feeding. The cartilage of the larynx is softer and its dimensions are approximately one-third that of an adult. In particular, the thyroid cartilage is more rounded and close to (and may overlap with) the hyoid bone. Within the larynx, the arytenoid cartilages are proportionately larger than the membranous portion of the true folds and appear bulky (Bluestone et al., 2003; Meyer et al., 1995). The length of the membranous portion of the vocal folds is approximately 1.3 to 2.0 millimeters (mm), with another 1 to 1.4 mm of cartilaginous portion (Hartnick & Bosley, 2008). Importantly, the respiratory epithelium that lines the larynx is mature but has a different distribution of ciliated epithelium and swells more easily (Meyer et al., 1995). The anterior to posterior distance of the pediatric glottic space is approximately 7 mm, with an approximate posterior width of 4 mm (Bluestone et al., 2003). The actual vocal folds comprise mostly the cartilaginous portion, favoring respiratory over phonatory function. At this time the subglottic region (within the ring of the cricoid) measures approximately 4 mm across. The trachea of an infant is approximately 4 cm in length and highly compliant, which can make it more prone to collapse. Within the digestive tract, the esophagus of a newborn functions with less precision than that of an older child or adult. Newborns are more prone to reflux and regurgitation, in part because the neural controls for peristalsis and the upper and lower esophageal sphincters (especially lower), are underdeveloped.

Within the first 2 to 3 years of life, there is considerable growth of the head and neck region. The skull enlarges and the larynx begins descending in the neck, lowering to cervical level C5 from C2–C3. The distance be-

tween the epiglottis and velum increases and the epiglottis begins to flatten from a more curled configuration. Cartilaginous structures harden and the hyoid bone ossifies. The cricoid cartilage loses some bulk and arytenoids reduce in their relative size to the rest of the glottis. The anatomic relationship of adult structures is generally in place in the child by age 6 to 7 years (Figure 2–2). Importantly, the microstructure of the vocal folds is beginning to differentiate from two to three layers of lamina propria (Hartnick & Bosley, 2008). There is continued growth of the larynx with increased weight and development of the child, and there is corresponding lowering of average fundamental frequency or pitch. These changes are gradual for both genders until the start of puberty. Throughout childhood, central and peripheral neural controls, along with the acquisition and mastery of speech and language skills, become more sophisticated.

During puberty, hormone-driven changes result in dramatic growth of the larynx, partic-

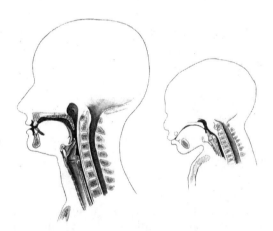

Figure 2–2. The adult larynx occupies a prominent position in the anterior neck. The cricoid ring lies approximately at the C-6 vertebral level. The cricoid ring in the young child is located at the C-4 vertebral level. From Myer, Cotton, & Schott, 1995. Reprinted with permission from Lippincott, Williams & Wilkins.

ularly in males, who will experience a significant increase in the prominence of the thyroid cartilage (commonly referred to as the Adam's apple). Throughout adulthood the angle of the thyroid cartilage in the female larynx remains flatter than that of same-aged males (Figure 2–3). In either gender, the position of the larynx in the neck descends to C6–C7. The membranous portions of the TVFs grow, reaching an adult length of 18 to 21 mm in males and 11 to 15 mm in females (Hirano, 1981). Moreover, the vocal fold layers as described above become more defined with age, reaching the full five layered histological composition around age 15 years (Hartnick & Bosley, 2008). For both genders, average fundamental frequencies lower for both genders, but the drop is especially striking for the peripubescent male. The rapid growth of the male larynx results in sudden, unexpected changes in pitch, referred to as pitch breaks. Across individuals, the rate and timeline of laryngeal growth and maturation vary, as does the rest of the pubertal changes and overall growth, but most young men's voices are sta-

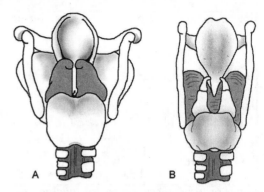

Figure 2–4. A. Posterior view of immature larynx and **B.** mature larynx. From *Voice Disorders* (2nd ed.) by C. Sapienza and B. Hoffman-Ruddy. Copyright © 2013 by Plural Publishing, Inc. Reprinted with permission.

ble by age 18 (Hollien, 2012) (see Figures 2–3 and 2–4).

Throughout adulthood, the laryngeal anatomy and physiology are relatively stable, with age-related changes occurring subtly and naturally over decades. In midlife and beyond, laryngeal changes can include ossification of the hyaline cartilages, weakening of the intrinsic muscles, thinning of the vocal fold cover, and changes to regional nerves and secretion-producing glands. Of course environmental, health, vocal use, and medical circumstances over the course of a lifetime can significantly impact vocal function later in life. Implications for diagnosis and treatment are discussed in later chapters.

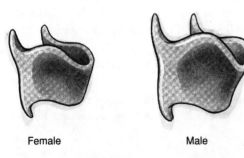

Female   Male

Figure 2–3. The female thyroid cartilage retains the rounded or gently angled appearance seen in the infant and young child. During puberty, the male thyroid cartilage laminae elongate and become acutely angled, causing the characteristic anterior prominence of the adult male thyroid cartilage. From Myer, Cotton, & Schott, 1995, p. 12. Reprinted with permission from Lippincott, Williams & Wilkins.

Anatomy and Physiology of the Upper Aerodigestive Tract

Nasal Passages

Function

The primary function of the nasal passages is to filter and humidify inspired air and house the sensory nerve endings for olfaction, but they also act as resonating cavities during voice and speech.

Structure and Spaces

The anterior aspect of the nasal passage is the nasal vestibule or the entrance to the nasal passage. The left and right nasal passages are separated by the septal cartilage. The lateral wall of each nasal passage has three lacey, bony protuberances called turbinates that extend into the nasal passage. Between the inferior, middle, and superior turbinates are corresponding meatuses or spaces. The entire nasal passage is covered with mucosal membranes that filter and humidify the inspired air. The uppermost or superior meatus contains the sensory nerve endings for cranial nerve I, the olfactory nerve.

The posterior portion of each nasal passage, (referred to as the choanae), opens into the nasopharynx. The boundaries of the nasopharynx are as follows: superior is the skull base, posterior is the posterior pharyngeal wall, and inferior is the velum (Figure 2–5). Important structures of the nasopharynx include the adenoids and the openings to the Eustachian tubes (torus tubaris).

Pharynx

Function

The pharynx extends from the level of the posterior nasal passages to the laryngeal vestibule and pharyngoesophageal segment (PES). It serves as a passage for both air and food and is the principal space of the vocal tract. Its muscles are configured to narrow, shorten, and lengthen the pharynx, which alters the resonating frequencies and thus the quality of the voice generated within the larynx. The pharynx is considered a fibromuscular tube with multiple layers of tissue ranging from

the outer mucosal lining to the deep buccopharyngeal fascia. In this deepest layer of the pharyngeal wall, there are multiple neural, circulatory, and lymphatic pathways (Moore, 1992).

Structure and Spaces

This muscular tube is bound at its superior aspect by the roof of the pharynx (or the skull base), at its posterior aspect by the posterior pharyngeal wall, and at its inferior aspect by the larynx and esophagus. Anterior boundaries differ depending on the corresponding pharyngeal "level." These functional levels include: the nasopharynx (posterior nasal openings), the oropharynx (oral cavity), and the laryngopharynx or hypopharynx (larynx and pyriform recesses).

The muscles responsible for narrowing the diameter of the pharynx during speech and swallowing are the pharyngeal constrictors. These striated muscles are arranged in a superior to inferior orientation and are so named (superior, middle, and inferior). The stylopharyngeus and suprahyoid muscles shorten and lift the laryngeal apparatus during speech and swallowing. The pharyngeal region is lined with primarily squamous cell epithelium and is richly innervated by cranial nerves IX, X, and XI. Table 2–2 lists the suprahyoid and pharyngeal muscles, attachments, and functions related to voice, speech, and swallowing.

Esophagus

Although it is entirely within the digestive tract, the esophagus is an important structure to include when reviewing anatomy and physiology pertaining to the voice. Located directly behind the trachea, the upper one-third of the esophagus comprises striated muscle, which transitions to smooth muscle in the lower or distal end. The uppermost

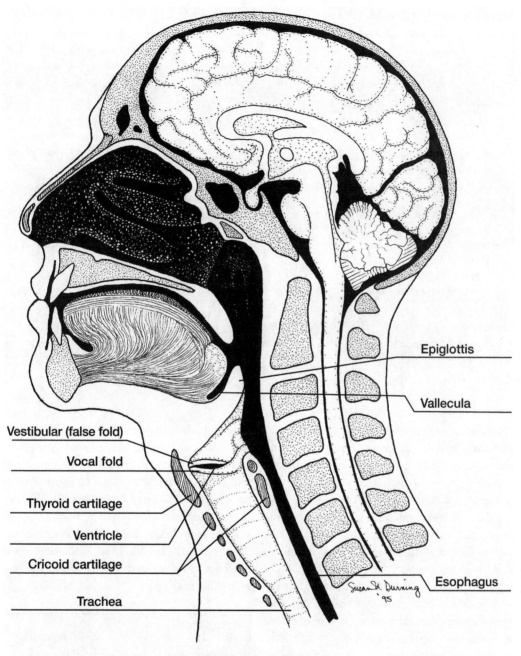

Epiglottis

Vallecula

Vestibular (false fold)

Vocal fold

Thyroid cartilage

Ventricle

Cricoid cartilage

Esophagus

Trachea

PHONATORY SYSTEM

Figure 2–5. Midsagittal view of the adult vocal tract; head and neck. Main structures labeled. From *Anatomy and Physiology Study Guide for Speech and Hearing* (2nd ed.) by W. Culbertson, S. Christensen, and D. Tanner. Copyright © 2012 by Plural Publishing, Inc. Reprinted with permission.

Table 2–2. Pharyngeal Muscles

Superior constrictor	Medial pterygoid plate; pterygomandibular raphe	Median pharyngeal raphe	Narrows the nasopharynx; weakest of the constrictor muscles
Middle constrictor	Hyoid bone	Median pharyngeal raphe	Narrows the oropharynx
Inferior constrictor	Lateral aspect of the thyroid laminae	Median pharyngeal raphe.	Narrows the hypopharynx; is the strongest of the constrictor muscles.
Pharyngoesophageal segment	Posterior cricoid	Circumferential, continuous fibers	Inferior aspect of the inferior constrictor; is a sphincter muscles that relaxes to open
Stylopharyngeus	Styloid process	Between the superior and middle constrictor to the thyroid cartilage	Raises the larynx; shortens the vertical length of the pharynx

sphincter and entrance to the esophagus is the PES, and its anterior attachment is to the posterior aspect of the cricoid cartilage. Other anatomic names frequently used interchangeably with the PES (though they do represent distinct anatomic differences having to do with muscle fiber type and orientation) are the upper esophageal sphincter (UES) and cricopharyngeus muscle (CP). A second sphincteric muscle (zone of high pressure in newborns) at the base of the esophagus where it enters the stomach is referred to as the lower esophageal sphincter (LES). Primarily a muscular conduit for food and liquids, under certain conditions digestive fluids (e.g., acids and pepsins, swallowed material) can be refluxed or regurgitated back up the esophagus to the region of the of the hypopharynx and posterior larynx. The presence of acidic material in these areas, particularly the posterior larynx, has significant implications for the health of the laryngeal and lower airway. In infants, the esophagus is approximately 8 to 10 cm long. The esophagus grows proportionately with the rest of the body and will reach an average length of 20 to 25 cm by adulthood (Murry & Carrau, 2006). Reflux or regurgitation during infancy is not uncommon (Allen, 2012; Campanozzi et al., 2009) and can be due to an underdeveloped digestive process, anatomy, or circumstances related to feeding.

Clinical Note: Excessive gastroesophageal or laryngopharyngeal reflux can result in serious airway injury regardless of one's age. It can present special airway and pulmonary health hazards for infants and young children. Symptoms of problematic reflux in an infant may include excessive crying, refusal to eat, hoarseness, and prolonged apnea.

Larynx

Function

The larynx is located at the intersection of the respiratory and digestive tracts and divides the lower and upper airway. As stated above, it performs three essential functions: It is part of the passageway for ventilation; it opens and closes or valves shut to protect the lower airway and permit increases in subglottic pressure for strain and lifting; and it is the sound generator for voice. Situated in the anterior neck, the larynx is suspended from the hyoid bone by the thyrohyoid membrane and ligament. At its most inferior aspect, the cricoid cartilage attaches to the upper part of the trachea by the cricotracheal membrane and ligament. Its inner covering is pseudostratified squamous cell epithelium.

Structure and Spaces

The larynx is comprised of skeletal components, musculature, and membranes. The spaces of the intrinsic or internal larynx are divided into functional levels. The glottis (rima glottidus) is the space between the TVFs when they are abducted or in an open position. The space just above the glottis is referred to as the supraglottis or supraglottic space, and just below is the subglottis or subglottic space. As one inspects the larynx using endoscopy, which is always a view from above, the typical appearance of the larynx reveals symmetrical right and left sides, each with mirror anatomic components and anterior and posterior regions. The anterior aspect of the larynx is referred to as the anterior commissure, and the posterior aspect is referred to as the posterior commissure or interarytenoid space. The visible components of the larynx include the TVFs; ventricular or false folds; arytenoid cartilages, aryepiglottic (AE) folds, and the epiglottis (Figure 2–6). The internal larynx receives its blood supply

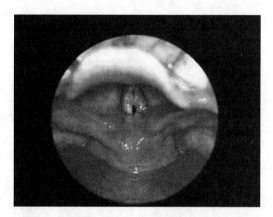

Figure 2–6. Larynx as viewed from above. Used with permission from the Center for Pediatric Voice Disorders, Cincinnati Children's Hospital Medical Center, Cincinnati, Ohio.

from the superior and inferior laryngeal arteries, each of which branch off the superior and inferior thyroid arteries, respectively. These arteries branch off the external carotid artery.

Laryngeal Skeleton

There are nine cartilages that make up the laryngeal apparatus, which is suspended from the hyoid bone by the thyrohyoid ligament and membrane. The horseshoe-shaped hyoid bone is the only unpaired bone in the body. Its bony prominences to which muscle and ligament attach are the greater and lesser cornuae. All cartilages of the larynx are comprised of hyaline tissue and ossify during adult life (Figures 2–7, 2–8, 2–9, and 2–10).

■ The **thyroid cartilage houses the vocal mechanism** and is the largest laryngeal cartilage. It has several distinguishing features, including two broad thyroid laminae, a thyroid notch, laryngeal prominence, and superior and inferior cornua (see Figure 2–10). In infants and young children, the laryngeal prominence is more rounded and flatter than that of an older child or adult.

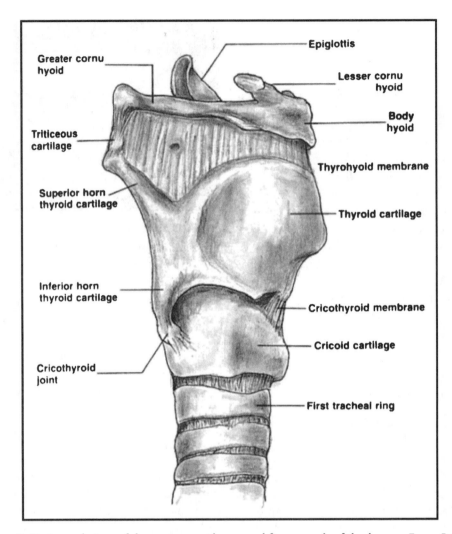

Figure 2–7. Lateral view of the major cartilages and framework of the larynx. From *Diagnosis and Treatment of Voice Disorders* by John S. Rubin, Robert T. Sataloff, and Gwen S. Korovin. Copyright © 2007 by Plural Publishing, Inc. Reprinted with permission.

■ The **cricoid cartilage** is a complete circumferential ring of cartilage that is the lowest cartilaginous structure of the laryngeal apparatus. It attaches to the thyroid cartilage by the cricothyroid membrane; and it attaches to the trachea below by the cricotracheal ligament and membrane. The anterior or front facing surface is narrow and is referred to as the arch of the cricoid; the posterior aspect is broad and its superior surface slopes downward. It has two arytenoid facets, on top of which each arytenoid sits.

The posterior aspect of the cricoid cartilage is broad and the anterior aspect is narrow. In the infant it is the cricoid cartilage that is more prominent, given its higher position.

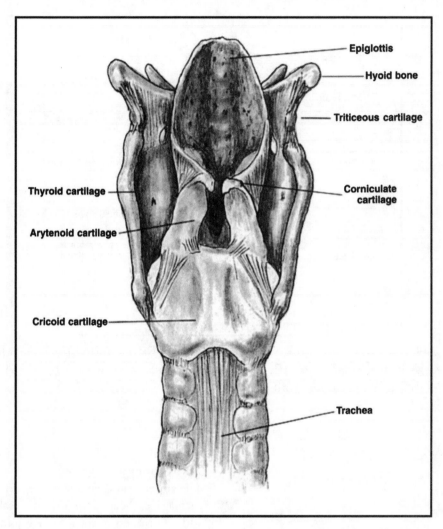

Figure 2–8. Posterior view of the laryngeal cartilages and framework. From *Diagnosis and Treatment of Voice Disorders* by John S. Rubin, Robert T. Sataloff, and Gwen S. Korovin. Copyright © 2007 by Plural Publishing, Inc. Reprinted with permission.

■ The **arytenoid cartilages** are paired cartilages, pyramidal in shape, that sit atop the posterior, sloping aspect of the superior surface of the cricoid cartilage known as the cricoid facets. Each arytenoid has three important features: the muscular process, the vocal process, and the apex (see Figure 2–10). The **vocal process** is where the vocal ligament attaches, thus it is always pointed toward the vocal fold. The **muscular process** is the broad posterior-lateral

aspect of the cartilage and is the place of attachment for the lateral and posterior cricoarytenoid muscles. The **apex** or uppermost tip of the cartilage provides structure and forms the base of the AE fold. The vocal ligament and the medial and lateral aspects of the thyroarytenoid muscle attach to the vocal process.

■ The **corniculate cartilage** sits atop the apex of the arytenoids adding height and aiding in posterior laryngeal closure through

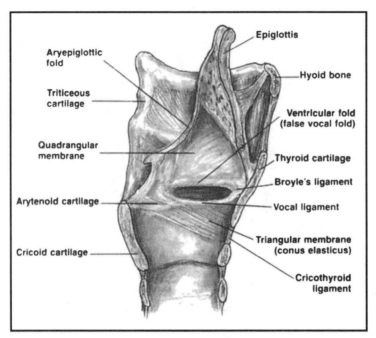

Figure 2–9. Laryngeal framework, sagittal section. From *Diagnosis and Treatment of Voice Disorders* by John S. Rubin, Robert T. Sataloff, and Gwen S. Korovin. Copyright © 2007 by Plural Publishing, Inc. Reprinted with permission.

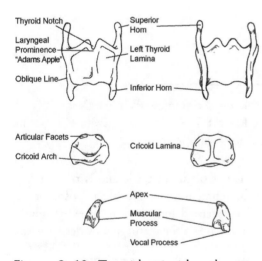

Figure 2–10. Thyroid, cricoid and arytenoid cartilages with major landmarks noted. From *Voice Disorders* (2nd ed.) by C. Sapienza and B. Hoffman-Ruddy. Copyright © 2013 by Plural Publishing, Inc. Reprinted with permission.

approximation with the petiole of the epiglottis during airway closure.

- The **cuneiform cartilage** is a separate, tiny cartilage embedded in the mucosal fold, adding firmness to the lower AE fold.

> In infants, the arytenoids are bulkier in proportion to the length of the vocal folds. Overall, the laryngeal cartilages are softer and will harden as the child ages (Figure 2–11).

- **Laryngeal Joints**
  - The two joints of the larynx are the cricothyroid and cricoarytenoid joints. Both are synovial joints with fibrous capsules (Moore, 1992). The cricothyroid facets and joints are located between the

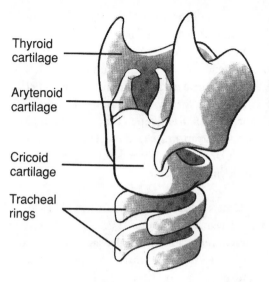

Thyroid cartilage

Arytenoid cartilage

Cricoid cartilage

Tracheal rings

Figure 2–11. Cartilage of the pediatric larynx and trachea, showing points of articulation of the thyroid with the lateral surface of the cricoid cartilage and also the articulation of the arytenoids with the posterior rim of the cricoid cartilage. The cricoid is a complete ring, in contrast to the tracheal cartilages, which are C-shaped. From Myer, Cotton, & Schott, 1995. Reprinted with permission from Lippincott, Williams & Wilkins.

Clinical Note: The cricoarytenoid joint, while small relative to other synovial joints, is subject to disarticulation, dislocation, fixation, and inflammatory systemic diseases such as rheumatoid arthritis.

depending on the muscular contractions of its attachments. The broader and rounded upper portion of the epiglottis is free to move and inverts during swallowing, thereby assisting in protection of the airway. The laryngeal surface of the epiglottis forms the anterior wall of the inner larynx, with its most narrow aspect attaching by the thyroepiglottic ligament to the inner and inferior aspect of the thyroid cartilage. Its upper aspect is broad and has a lingual (faces toward the tongue base) surface and laryngeal (faces toward the larynx) surface. It attaches to the hyoid bone by way of the hyoepiglottic ligament. The space between the lingual surface and the tongue base is known as the vallecula(e). This space is split into a left and right side by the glossoepiglottic fold. At the narrow base of the laryngeal surface of the epiglottis, there is a prominence

lateral aspect of the cricoid cartilage and the inferior horn of the thyroid cartilage. The presence of these joints permits the thyroid cartilage to tilt forward during contraction of the cricothyroid muscles.

The cricoarytenoid joint has a range of motion that is accomplished by contraction of the various intrinsic muscles in conjunction with the mechanics of the joint (Moore & von Leden, 1961). Attachment of the arytenoid cartilage to the cricoid cartilage is by way of the cricoarytenoid ligament. The mobility of this joint permits tilting, sliding, and rotation of the arytenoids.

The **epiglottis** is a separate and flexible shoehorn-shaped cartilage that shifts position

Clinical Note: In anyone, but particularly infants and young children, the cricoid cartilage is the narrowest portion of the airway. When there is trauma or infection in that region, the overlying respiratory epithelium can become inflamed and swell, further narrowing the airway. Croup is one common inflammatory condition that can narrow the subglottic airway and cause a distinct sound during a cough, often described as a barking seal sound. Severe croup can create an airway emergency.

called the tubercle or petiole of the epiglottis. In infants and young children, the epiglottic tip often has an "omega" shape to it. In a very young child, the tip of the epiglottis can sometimes be seen during an oral-motor exam.

Laryngeal Muscles

The muscles of the larynx are categorized by both their location (intrinsic and extrinsic) and function. The extrinsic muscles are described as either laryngeal elevators or depressors, while the intrinsic muscles are cross-categorized as tensors or relaxers, abductors or adductors. All the muscles of the larynx are striated, and the name of each muscle often describes its origin and insertion. Direction of contraction is typically toward a muscle's point of origin.

Extrinsic Muscles. The external laryngeal muscles include the large, paired strap muscles of the neck that either elevate or lower the entire larynx within the neck. Table 2–3 displays the external strap muscles by whether they elevate or lower the larynx (Figures 2–12 and 2–13). Remember that the external laryngeal/strap muscles are deep to (or under) the platysma, the broad thin muscle of the neck and lower face.

Intrinsic Muscles. The intrinsic muscles of the larynx are so named because both of their attachments are within the laryngeal apparatus. They serve to shorten or lengthen; tense and/or relax; or abduct (open) or adduct (close) the TVFs. With the exception of the transverse interarytenoid muscle, all intrinsic muscles are paired. Table 2–4 presents each muscle group; origin and insertion and action

Table 2–3. Extrinsic Laryngeal Muscles

Muscle	Origin	Insertion	Action
Suprahyoid muscles			
Anterior/posterior bellies of digastricus	Anterior: fossa of the mandible Posterior: temporal bone	Intermediate tendon Intermediate tendon and hyoid bone	Stabilizes and raises the hyoid during speech and swallowing
Mylohyoid	Inner rim of the mandible	Median raphe	Raises hyoid during speech and swallowing
Stylohyoid	Styloid process of temporal bone	Hyoid bone	Raises and retracts the hyoid and hyolaryngeal complex during speech and swallowing
Geniohyoid	Inner front rim of the mandible	Hyoid bone	Assists in raising the hyolaryngeal complex; pulling it up and forward
Hyoglossus	Hyoid bone	Lateral tongue	Lowers the back of the tongue

Table 2–3. *continued*

Muscle	Origin	Insertion	Action
Infrahyoid muscles			
Sternohyoid	Manubrium of the sternum	Hyoid bone	Lowers the larynx
Thyrohyoid	Lateral thyroid laminae; oblique line	Hyoid bone	Shortens the distance between the thyroid cartilage and hyoid bone
Sternothyroid	Manubrium of the sternum	Hyoid bone	Contracts in the direction of origin, lowering the larynx
Omohyoid	Inferior belly: scapula Superior belly: intermediate tendon	Intermediate tendon Hyoid bone	Lowers the larynx

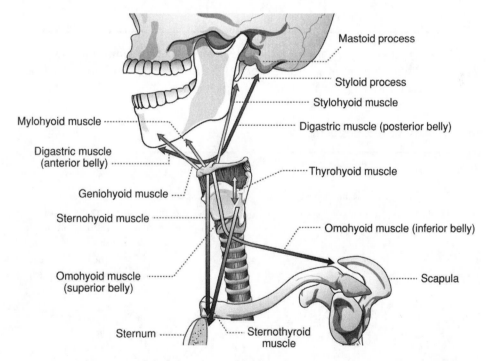

Figure 2–12. Schematic of the direction of action for the extrinsic (supra and infrahyoid) laryngeal muscles. From *Speech and Voice Science* (2nd ed.) by A. Behrman. Copyright © 2013 by Plural Publishing, Inc. Reprinted with permission.

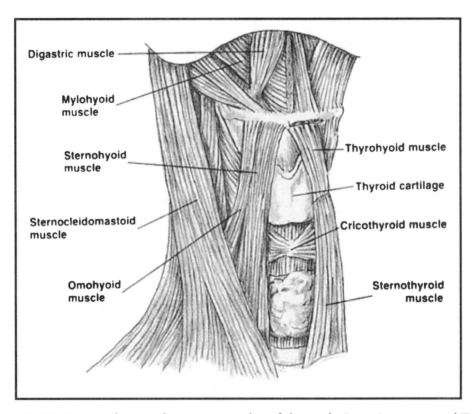

Figure 2–13. Extrinsic laryngeal or strap muscles of the neck. From *Diagnosis and Treatment of Voice Disorders* by John S. Rubin, Robert T. Sataloff, and Gwen S. Korovin. Copyright © 2007 by Plural Publishing, Inc. Reprinted with permission.

Table 2–4. Intrinsic Muscles of the Larynx

Muscle	Origin	Insertion	Action
Posterior cricoarytenoid	Medial aspect of the posterior cricoid	Lateral aspect of the muscular process of the arytenoid cartilage	Rotates the vocal process of the arytenoids out and elevates the tip, elongates the vocal fold; is the only muscle to **abduct** the vocal folds.
Lateral cricoarytenoid	Antero-lateral aspect of the cricoid	Medial aspect of the muscular process of the arytenoid cartilage	Rotates and lowers the vocal process of the arytenoids midline, lowering and elongating the vocal folds; **adducts** the vocal folds

Table 2–4. *continued*

Muscle	Origin	Insertion	Action
Interarytenoids			
■ Transverse	Muscular process of the arytenoid	Muscular process of the opposite arytenoid	Both the unpaired transverse and paired obliques draw the arytenoid bases medially, adducting the TVFs
■ Oblique	Muscular process of the arytenoid	Apex of the opposite arytenoid	
Thyroarytenoid			The vocalis muscle lowers, thickens, and shortens the vocal fold and is considered a **tensor**; the lateral or muscularis portion is considered a **relaxer**.
■ Medial (vocalis)	Inner angle of the thyroid laminae	Vocal process of the arytenoid (medial and lateral)	
■ Lateral (muscularis)			
Cricothyroid			When contracted, the CT pulls the thyroid laminae down and forward, thus lowering and lengthening the vocal folds, and so is considered a **tensor**.
■ Pars recta	Anterior aspect of the cricoid cartilage	The lower margin of the thyroid lamina; pars recta has a more vertical orientation; pars oblique, a more angled orientation.	
■ Pars oblique			

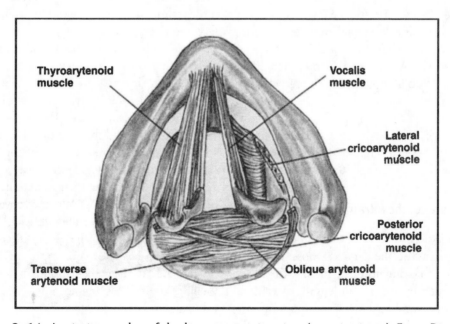

Figure 2–14. Intrinsic muscles of the larynx, superior view (anterior is up). From *Diagnosis and Treatment of Voice Disorders* by John S. Rubin, Robert T. Sataloff, and Gwen S. Korovin. Copyright © 2007 by Plural Publishing, Inc. Reprinted with permission.

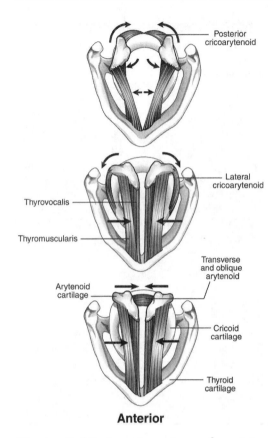

Figure 2–15. Superior view of activity of the intrinsic laryngeal muscles, anterior is down. From *Speech and Voice Science* (2nd ed.) by A. Behrman. Copyright © 2013 by Plural Publishing, Inc. Reprinted with permission.

(Figures 2–14 through 2–19 depict the location, position, and function of these muscles).

Structures of the Intrinsic Larynx

Vocal Folds. The TVFs are the vibrating mechanism of the larynx whose composition is three-dimensional, in that they have height/depth, width, and length. Over time, the term "vocal fold" replaced the term "vocal cord," as it more accurately represents the multidimensional, multilayered structural design of the anatomy. Along their lengthwise

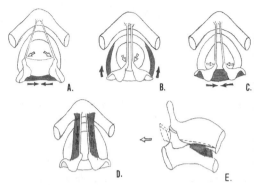

Figure 2–16. Action of the intrinsic laryngeal muscles, anterior is up. From *Diagnosis and Treatment of Voice Disorders* by John S. Rubin, Robert T. Sataloff, and Gwen S. Korovin. Copyright © 2007 by Plural Publishing, Inc. Reprinted with permission.

dimension, the TVFs are described as having a membranous (or soft tissue) portion and a cartilaginous portion (attachment to and including the vocal process of the arytenoid). The vibrating surface of the vocal fold edge is mostly along its medial edge. The lateral surface is adjacent to the ventricle (Figure 2–20). In a coronal view of the vocal fold, it is possible to appreciate that there is a lower and upper lip to the medial edge. This anatomic arrangement is not always appreciated from the typical endoscopic view (Figure 2–21).

First described by Minoru Hirano in 1977, the membranous portion of the TVFs can be partitioned as "cover," "transition," and "body" based on their functions during phonation. Histologically, the "cover" includes the epithelium and superficial lamina propria, "transition" includes the intermediate and deep layers of lamina propria (comprising the vocal ligament); and the "body" includes the thyroarytenoid muscle. The vocal ligament is also considered the upper free edge of the conus elasticus, a sheath of elastic membrane (part of the cricothyroid ligament) that extends up to the vocal ligament from

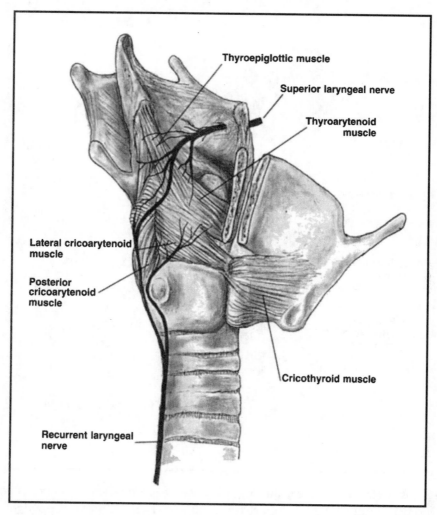

Figure 2–17. Intrinsic laryngeal muscles, lateral view. From *Diagnosis and Treatment of Voice Disorders* by John S. Rubin, Robert T. Sataloff, and Gwen S. Korovin. Copyright © 2007 by Plural Publishing, Inc. Reprinted with permission.

the cricoid cartilage. Each layer of the "cover" of the vocal fold has a discrete composition. The later section on vocal fold histology will provide an in-depth discussion of these important anatomic distinctions. The microstructure of the TVFs is significant for the physiology of phonation and the impact and diagnosis of TVF lesions (Figures 2–22 and 2–23).

Ventricular Folds, Vestibular Ligament, and Quadrangular Membrane. A second set of folds referred to as the "false" or ventricular (or vestibular) vocal folds are positioned just superior and lateral to the true folds, also extending from the thyroid cartilage to the arytenoid cartilages. Each is composed of mucous membrane, fibroelastic membrane, fat, and some muscle fibers. Contained in the

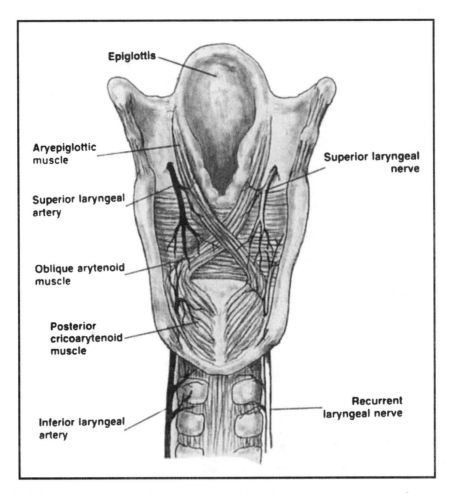

Figure 2–18. Instrinsic laryngeal muscles, posterior view. From *Diagnosis and Treatment of Voice Disorders* by John S. Rubin, Robert T. Sataloff, and Gwen S. Korovin. Copyright © 2007 by Plural Publishing, Inc. Reprinted with permission.

ventricular folds are the vestibular ligaments. Vestibular ligaments are the free edges and inferior aspects of the quadrangular membrane. This submucosal connective tissue extends from the arytenoids to the epiglottis. Between the true and false folds is a space referred to as the laryngeal ventricle. This space, again not always visible during examination, contains mucus-secreting glands that help moisten the surface of the folds, thus reducing friction during phonation. The ventricular folds can be approximated through compression, par-

ticularly during airway protection, straining, and cough. They are less resistant to the outflow of air from the lungs and can be set into motion during phonation. However, during normal phonation, these folds do not vibrate as an independent source of sound (Figure 2–24). Strobe samples 7 and 10 on the DVD demonstrate supraglottic and ventricular fold voicing.

Aryepiglottic Folds. Forming the lateral walls of the larynx and thus separating the

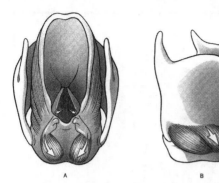

Figure 2–19. A. Contraction of the posterior cricoarytenoid muscle (sole abductor) causes abduction of the vocal folds away from midline. **B.** Contraction of the cricothyroid muscle causes the thyroid laminae to tip forward and down, lengthening the true vocal folds and the dimension of the anterior–posterior dimension of the larynx. Adapted from Myer, Cotton, & Schott, 1995. Reprinted with permission from Lippincott, Williams & Wilkins.

intrinsic larynx from the hypopharynx, the AE folds are composed of mucosal membrane and fibroelastic tissue that extend from the tip of the arytenoids to the lateral edge of the epiglottis. Within these folds of tissue

are the AE muscle fibers, extensions of the oblique interarytenoid muscles. Contraction of the AE muscles aid in pulling the epiglottis downward.

Vocal Fold Microstructure

Contributed by Keiko Ishikawa

Understanding the microstructure of the vocal folds is key to understanding vocal fold health, vocal fold pathologies, and phonation. In the following section you are provided a "primer" of vocal fold histology, starting with the basics. The primer is followed by an

Phonation

Inspiration

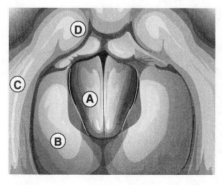 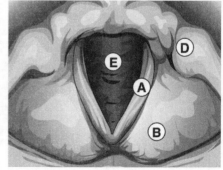

Figure 2–20. Superior view of the glottis; anterior is down. Vocal folds adducted on left and abducted on right. (A) True vocal fold, (B) ventricular fold, (C) aryepiglottic fold, (D) arytenoid, and (E) glottis. From *Speech and Voice Science* (2nd ed.) by A. Behrman. Copyright © 2013 by Plural Publishing, Inc. Reprinted with permission.

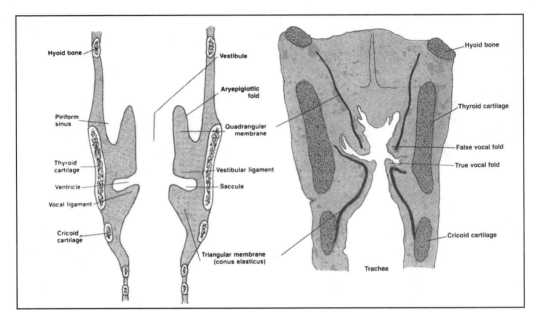

Figure 2–21. The human larynx, vocal folds, ventricle and ventricular folds presented in a coronal view. From *Diagnosis and Treatment of Voice Disorders* by John S. Rubin, Robert T. Sataloff, and Gwen S. Korovin. Copyright © 2007 by Plural Publishing, Inc. Reprinted with permission.

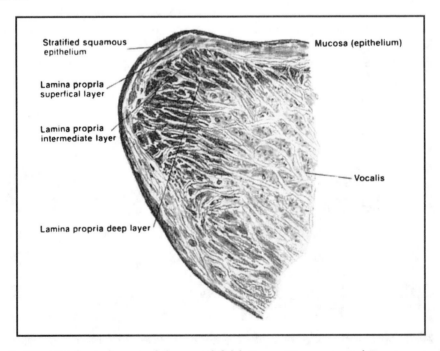

Figure 2–22. Histologic layers of the vocal fold. From *Diagnosis and Treatment of Voice Disorders* by John S. Rubin, Robert T. Sataloff, and Gwen S. Korovin. Copyright © 2007 by Plural Publishing, Inc. Reprinted with permission.

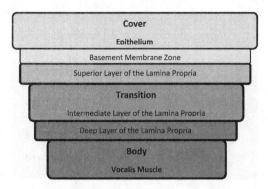

Figure 2–23. Graphic depiction of the layers of the vocal fold; body and cover relationship.

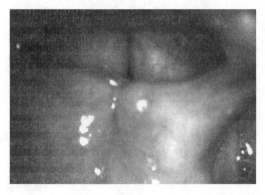

Figure 2–24. Endoscopic image of ventricular or false fold phonation. Used with permission from Center for Pediatric Voice Disorders, Cincinnati Children's Hospital Medical Center, Cincinnati, Ohio.

in-depth description of the microstructure of the vocal fold in children and adults, as it is currently understood.

Basics of Histology

Histology is a branch of biological science that studies how cells and other microscopic structures in tissue optimize function of an organ. Fundamentally, histological studies examine thinly sliced tissue under a microscope, and the tissue is chemically treated to highlight structures of interest. Histological techniques have been widely used in vocal fold research and have provided a foundation for our current understanding of voice production and pathology. In order to discuss histology of the vocal folds, it would be helpful to know the basics of histology. Therefore, a brief introduction to histology is presented below.

The human body is made of four types of tissue: epithelial, connective, muscular, and nervous. The mucosal lining of the larynx is made up of these tissue types. Epithelial tissue, or epithelium, is the outer covering of an organ. In general, epithelial tissue is classified based on the shape and arrangement of the epithelial cells. There are four basic types of epithelial cells: squamous, cuboidal, columnar, and transitional. Squamous cells are flat like a sheet; cuboidal cells have approximately the same height and width, like a box; and columnar cells are tall and shaped like a column, as the name suggests. Squamous cells are also categorized into keratinized and nonkeratinized types. The keratinized type is seen in the skin where desiccation from water loss needs to be prevented. Mucosa are nonkeratinized because water loss is less of an issue (Mescher, 2010). Transitional cells are dome-like and found only in the bladder.

The arrangement of epithelial cells is categorized in three ways: simple, stratified, and pseudostratified. In simple epithelium, the cells are arranged in one layer, while stratified epithelium is made of multiple layers of epithelial cells. In pseudostratified epithelium, all cells are also arranged in one layer—however, they *appear* to be in multiple layers because the cells are tall and interwoven. The look of this cell arrangement is the reason that this type of epithelium is referred to as *pseudo*stratified.

Connective tissue has many different forms, including bone, cartilage, blood, adipose tissue, loose connective tissue, dense connective tissue, and specialized connective tissue. The connective tissue in the vocal fold is considered to be loose connective tissue. Another type of vocal fold connective tissue is the basement membrane zone (BMZ). This specialized connective tissue is just beneath the epithelium. The BMZ provides an anchoring site for the epithelium and underlying connective tissue. The BMZ plays an important role in wound healing, as it provides a scaffold for cells to migrate to the injury site.

Despite the wide variety of tissue types, all connective tissues have a common embryonic origin, mesenchyme, which is one of the three primary embryonic tissues. Connective tissue is composed of cells and extracellular matrix (ECM). The ECM consists of protein fibers and ground substance. The composition of cells, fibers, and ground substance varies among the different types of connective tissue, and this variety gives rise to wide structural diversity. The ECM was once thought to merely provide structural support for the tissue, but it is now well known that the ECM also signals cells for executing multiple biological functions, such as survival, migration, proliferation, and differentiation of cells (Alberts et al., 2002).

Ground substance is a gel-like material that surrounds protein fibers of the ECM. This gel helps the tissue resist compressive forces by acting as a shock absorber (Alberts et al., 2002). It also participates in various biological activities, including transport of nutrients, metabolites, and hormones from the blood to tissue cells. Ground substance is composed of glycosaminoglycans (GAGs) and adhesive glycoproteins. GAGs are classified into five categories based on their chemical compositions: (1) hyaluronan or hyaluronic acid, (2) dermatan sulfate, (3) chondroitin sulfate, (4) keratan sulfate, and (5) heparin sulfate. The difference in their chemistry determines their biological roles in the tissue. Hyaluronic acid is the primary type of GAG that determines water content of the tissue (Alberts et al., 2002).

Vocal Fold Histology

Our current understanding of vocal fold microstructure and its relation to vocal physiology is built upon Hirano's histological studies from the 1970s. Hirano was the first to relate the microstructure to vibratory characteristics of the vocal fold. His histological observations led to the development of the body-cover theory of voice production, which continues to be the foundation of voice research and clinical practice today. Hirano's work was expanded by Gray, who examined constituents of the ECM beyond fibrous proteins. Great strides were made in biochemical characterization of these ECM molecules and their relation to biomechanics and pathology of the vocal fold. As the technologies in biomedical science advanced, researchers began applying new molecular techniques to study interactions between the cells and ECM in various physiological processes. At present, molecular biology of the vocal fold is one of the most rapidly growing areas of voice science, and we have begun to understand how cells, proteins, and genes in the vocal fold tissue work. The following section will provide a histological description of the adult vocal fold based on representative works in this area.

Recall that the vocal fold is *composed* of three types of tissue: epithelial, connective, and muscular, but *histologically* the adult vocal fold is *divided* into five layers (Hirano, 1977). The outermost layer is epithelial tissue. Deep to the epithelial tissue is connective tissue called lamina propria. The lamina propria has three layers; superficial, intermediate, and deep lamina propria (SLP, ILP, and DLP). The innermost layer of the vocal fold is muscular tissue—more specifically, the thyrovocalis muscle (see Figure 2–22).

Epithelial Tissue

The epithelial tissue of the TVF is nonkeratinized stratified squamous epithelium (Gray, 2000). It is different from surrounding epithelial tissue in the larynx (i.e., regions above and below the vocal folds), which is classified as pseudostratified ciliated columnar epithelium. In general, stratified squamous epithelium is found in the body where the tissue is required to withstand mechanical stress. When considering that the vocal fold tissue is constantly under mechanical stress from phonation, it makes sense that the vocal fold is covered by this type of epithelium.

In addition to protecting against mechanical stress, the epithelium provides a barrier between the inner and outer environment. The epithelium executes this function by selectively transporting ions and molecules across the membrane. One of the barrier functions relevant to vocal health is to prevent desiccation of the vocal fold tissue. Drying the surface of the vocal fold increases viscosity and stiffness of the tissue (Hemler, Wieneke, Lebacq, & Dejonckere, 2001) and results in a change in voice quality (Hemler, Wieneke, & Dejonckere, 1997). Phonation with dry vocal fold surfaces could thus require greater phonatory effort, increasing risk of vocal fold injury. These findings and clinical observations led researchers to focus on the role of the epithelium in maintenance of vocal fold hydration. It has been shown that vocal fold epithelium is equipped with several mechanisms that help regulate and maintain the hydration level of the vocal fold surface, including: the sodium-potassium ($Na+K+ATPase$) pump, sodium-potassium-chloride ($Na+K+2Cl-$) cotransporter, epithelial sodium channels (ENaC), cystic fibrosis transmembrane regulator (CFTR) chloride channels, and aquaporin (AQP) water channels in the vocal fold epithelium (Leydon, Sivasankar, Falciglia, Atkins, & Fisher, 2009).

Lamina Propria

The vocal fold tissue is composed of cells and extracellular materials. But the three layers of the lamina propria differ in their cellular and extracellular composition (Catten, Gray, Hammond, Zhou, & Hammond, 1998; Hammond, Gray, Butler, Zhou, & Hammond, 1998; Hartnick, Rehbar, & Prasad, 2005; Hirano, 1977; Madruga de Melo et al., 2003; Newman, Butler, Hammond, & Gray, 2000). The density, type, and arrangement of cells and extracellular fibers affect mechanical properties of the vocal fold tissue (Gray, Titze, Chan, & Hammond, 1999; Hirano, 1977). Therefore, the difference in biochemical composition among the three layers of the lamina propria is an important factor to consider when examining vibratory characteristics of the vocal fold. The SLP is characterized by the presence of loose fibrous proteins; the ILP is identified by abundance of elastic fibers; and the DLP is represented by dense collagen fibers. It is believed that collagen fibers play a role in maintaining organization of the vocal folds, and elastic fibers help rapidly restore the vocal folds to their original form during phonation. The loose fibrous proteins of the SLP make it the most pliable layer of the lamina propria. The pliability becomes less in the ILP and the least in the DLP. This difference in the mechanical properties among the layers is the premise of the cover-body theory.

You have already learned that the cover consists of the epithelium and SLP; the transition consists of ILP and DLP; and the body consists of the thyrovocalis muscle. The cover is often referred to as the vibratory portion of the vocal folds. The greater pliability of the cover allows it to ride on the body during phonation and makes it the main part of the vocal fold that controls glottic pulses during phonation. Structural integrity of the cover is crucial for healthy voice production. However, the cover is more vulnerable to injury not only because it is the first site that absorbs the mechanical stress, but also its high pliability allows it to vibrate in much greater amplitude than the body during phonation. The pliability of the cover can be significantly altered by injury or biochemical changes. For example, a scarred vocal fold becomes stiffer than a normal vocal fold. Likewise, vocal fold edema induced by hormonal changes or inflammation can also increase stiffness of the cover (Titze, 1994). These changes in the cover change how it is able to vibrate and can result in some degree of dysphonia.

Clinical Note: The SLP is also referred to as *Reinke's space.* Accumulation of extracellular fluid in this layer occurs in reaction to trauma or inflammation. Reinke edema is a common etiology across adulthood (young and older) and is associated with disturbances of voice.

Developmental Changes in the Vocal Fold Across the Lifespan

This section is a review of how the microstructure of the vocal folds changes over the course of the lifespan. Clinicians in pediatric voice care are uniquely challenged by voice changes that accompany physical growth of a child. As mentioned earlier, the size and proportion of laryngeal framework, size of the vocal fold, and position of the larynx changes during development (Figures 2–25 and 2–26). Size and position are not the only aspects of the larynx that change during development. The microstructure of the vocal fold tissue also changes with age. Understanding these changes that occur during development is important because they account for the biological basis of vocal maturation.

Recall that ground substance is a gel-like material in the connective tissue that is made of several different types of GAGs and adhesive glycoproteins. Ground substance in the vocal fold lamina propria plays multiple roles in maintaining health of the vocal fold tissue. One of the GAGs, hyaluronic acid, is involved in regulation of tissue viscosity, filling of the extracellular space, and absorption of mechanical stress from phonation (Ward, Thibeault, & Gray, 2002). It is also believed that hyaluronic acid plays a significant role in wound healing; therefore, maintaining optimal level of hyaluronic acid may be important for prevention of scarring after vocal fold injury (Thibeault, Gray, Bless, Chan, & Ford, 2002).

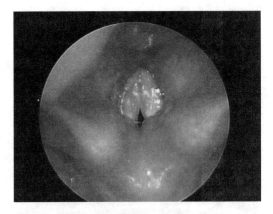

Figure 2–25. Endoscopic image of a pediatric larynx (*anterior is up*). Used with permission from Center for Pediatric Voice Disorders, Cincinnati Children's Hospital Medical Center, Cincinnati, Ohio.

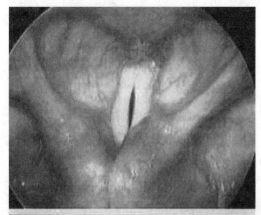

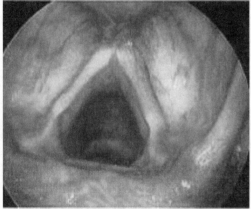

Figure 2–26. Endoscopic image of an older adult larynx (*anterior is up*) depicting age related changes. Used with permission from Center for Pediatric Voice Disorders, Cincinnati Children's Hospital Medical Center, Cincinnati, Ohio.

Fetus and Infant

There are several morphological features unique to fetal and infant vocal folds. The mucosa of the newborn vocal fold is thicker relative to the length compared with that of the adult vocal fold. The mucosa of the newborn vocal fold also lacks the vocal ligament, and the layers of the lamina propria are not clearly defined (Hirano, Kurita, & Nakashima, 1983). The uniform distribution of ECM constituents in the lamina propria has

been confirmed by multiple studies (Prades et al., 2010; Sato, Hirano, & Nakashima, 2001; Schweinfurth & Thibeault, 2008); however, one report observed the vocal ligament in fetal vocal folds (Nita et al., 2009). This discrepancy between the studies may be due to methodological differences. The monolayer lamina propria structure is also present in fetal vocal folds (Buhler et al., 2008; Rosenberg & Schweinfurth, 2009). This one-layer structure of the infant vocal fold was also based on the cellular distribution in the lamina propria (Hartnick et al., 2005). Cell density is significantly higher in the fetal and infant lamina propria than in the adult lamina propria (Hirano et al., 1983; Rosenberg & Schweinfurth, 2009), and the density may begin decreasing as early as 27 weeks of gestation (Rosenberg & Schweinfurth). Based on the striking difference in the layer structure between the vocal folds of infants and adults, researchers have theorized that mechanical stress from postpartum phonation drives the development of the three-layer structure of the lamina propria.

Young Children

The vocal folds of young children do not have the three-layer lamina propria structure as seen in adults (Hartnick et al., 2005; Hirano et al., 1983). The timing for emergence of the three-layer lamina propria structure has not been well defined. It has been reported that the immature ligament develops by the age of 4, suggesting the emergence of the layer structure (Hirano et al., 1983). Two distinct layers of cellular populations have been observed as early as 2 months of age, suggesting the beginning of a bilayer of structure development (Hartnick et al., 2005). It has been reported that the early cellular differentiation of the three lamina propria layers appears at about 7 years of age, yet the fully differentiated fiber composition seen in the adult three-layer structure appears much later, around the age of 12 to 13 years.

Adolescents

Adolescence is a unique period in voice development. The voice matures, and a clear difference between male and female voices emerges. It has been hypothesized that the voice change is due not only to the growth of the vocal fold and laryngeal framework, but also to the microstructural changes in the vocal fold tissue. This theory has been supported by several studies. As mentioned earlier, the histological studies have reported that the three-layer structure develops in mid-adolescence (Hirano et al., 1983), and this change appears to begin around 13 years of age (Hartnick et al., 2005). It appears that gender-specific vocal fold microstructure begins to emerge during adolescence. Newman et al. (2000) observed the intergender difference in collagen content of the lamina propria in adult and geriatric vocal folds, but not in infant vocal folds. It has also been hypothesized that the structural changes are driven by sex hormones. This hypothesis has been tested by searching for sex hormone receptors in the vocal fold tissue; however, findings have been inconsistent (Nacci et al., 2011; Newman, Butler, Hammond, & Gray, 2000; Schneider et al., 2007; Voelter et al., 2008). The inconsistency has been attributed to differences in histological techniques and interpretation of the results.

Older Adult and Elderly

Vocal fold tissue undergoes morphological changes due to aging. A number of studies have documented these changes. The male and female vocal folds age differently (Hirano, Kurita, & Sakaguchi, 1989). The SLP becomes more edematous with age in both genders; however, thickening of the vocal fold cover is more evident in females. The older male vocal fold is characterized by overall thinning and atrophy of elastic fibers in the ILP, along with thickening of the DLP with increased density of collagen fibers. Age-related change is also observed in the DLP. In males, collagen fibers increase in their size and density, and their arrangement becomes more random. This arrangement is in contrast with the fibers in the young vocal fold, which run parallel to the edge of the fold. These changes are not significant among females (Hirano et al., 1983). A more recent study evaluated change in thickness of the lamina propria and epithelial cell density (Ximenes Filho, Tsuji, do Nascimento, & Sennes, 2003). Thinning of the lamina propria was observed in both genders in this study, with greater changes in males. Epithelial density decreased with age in both genders, again with greater changes in males.

The age-related changes in the distribution of elastic fibers in the ILP are not well understood. Hirano and his colleagues reported that elastic fibers atrophy and their density decreases in males after the age of 40 (Hirano et al., 1983). Arrangement of elastic fibers in the SLP was examined in a later study by the same group, which reported that the fibers in the aged vocal folds were arranged less orderly and formed more complicated networks compared with those of younger adults (Sato & Hirano, 1997). On the contrary, a more recent study by Hammond and Gray (1998) reported that the distribution of elastin, a protein that composes elastic fibers, appears to increase with age. Hammond and Gray attributed this discrepancy to a possible change in elastic fiber formation caused by a decrease in elastin turnover, as well as methodological differences.

Age-related changes occur not only in lamina propria but also in the thyrovocalis muscle. Muscle fibers of the thyrovocalis muscle are much thinner in newborns compared with adults. As aging progresses, the fibers become atrophied. Clinically, elderly patients often present with presbylarynx, which is characterized by bowing of the vocal fold (Stemple, Glaze, & Klaben, 2000). This is likely a result of the atrophy of the thyrovocalis muscle and thinning of SLP. It is also known that the average fundamental frequency of the male speaking voice is higher in older individuals (Hollien & Shipp, 1972). This phenomenon is likely due to a decrease in the vocal fold mass from the atrophy and thinning. Knowledge of the microstructure of the vocal folds and how it changes over time is important for understanding concepts related to normal phonatory function, abnormal conditions (e.g., presence of lesions and/or misuse) and their assessment and subsequent treatment. Appendix A provides the reader with an in-depth review of wound healing as it relates to vocal fold microstructure.

Pediatric Respiratory Anatomy and Physiology

This section explains the anatomic structures and the physiologic processes for breathing during voice production. Most speech sounds produced by humans are produced during exhalation of air from the lungs. Vibration of the vocal folds depends on a sufficient, continuous stream of air during the expiratory phase of breathing. One must not forget that the physiologic purpose of breathing is primarily for oxygen and carbon dioxide exchange for sustaining life function. We are limited in the length of phrases (singing or speaking) and the intensity at which we produce voicing by the need to maintain a consistent, sufficient exchange of gases. Muscles in the thoracic and abdominal areas are essential for breathing, and these muscles and their role in the physiologic process are explained.

Anatomy and Physiology of the Lower Respiratory Tract

Tracheal Airway

Function

When we take a breath in, we bring air initially through our upper airway. The upper airway is generally defined as the nose, mouth, pharynx, and larynx. Air passes through the vocal folds in the larynx down to the lower airway, which consists of the trachea, bronchi/bronchioles, and the lungs (Figure 2–27). Exchange of air gases occurs across the capillary membrane in the alveoli of the lungs, and the process for breathing out air follows the same pathway in the opposite direction.

Structures and Spaces

The trachea is a structure made up of a series of 16 to 20 incomplete or C-shaped cartilaginous

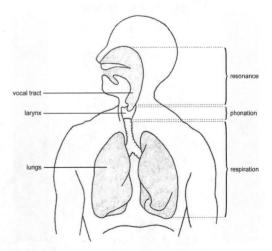

Figure 2–27. Respiratory and upper vocal tract. From *Clinical Voice Pathology. Theory and Management* (4th ed.) by Joseph Stemple, Leslie Glaze, and Bernice K. Klaben. Copyright © 2010 by Plural Publishing, Inc. Reprinted with permission.

rings. These rings are horizontally oriented with the incomplete portion adjacent to the esophagus. In this posterior location, the trachealis muscle (refer back to Figure 2–11) attaches to the ends of the tracheal cartilage. Between each cartilage ring is tracheal membrane. The combination of the support of the cartilage, membrane, and the flexibility of the smooth trachealis muscles allows the trachea to adapt and not collapse with the changing pressures that occur during normal breathing and speech production. At its uppermost or superior end, the trachea connects to the larynx by way of the cricotracheal membrane and ligament. At its most inferior aspect, it bifurcates and becomes the right and left mainstem bronchi (Figure 2–28). The location of the split is referred to as the carina. The trachea is lined with pseudostratified, ciliated, columnar epithelium. The lining also contains some goblet cells that secrete mucus. The cilia embedded in the epithelium perform an important function in that they move mucus and any foreign material up out of the lower airway.

> Clinical Note: *Intubation.* When an infant or child needs assistance with respiration, an intubation tube may be needed to facilitate artificial ventilator support. An intubation procedure involves the placement of an endotracheal tube through the nose or mouth, the pharynx, down between the vocal folds into the trachea. There are several potential risks from intubation, including post-intubation croup and subglottic stenosis. Complications may also occur from difficult intubation procedures involving multiple attempts, coughing around the tube, and prolonged placement.

Bronchi, Bronchial Tree, and Lungs

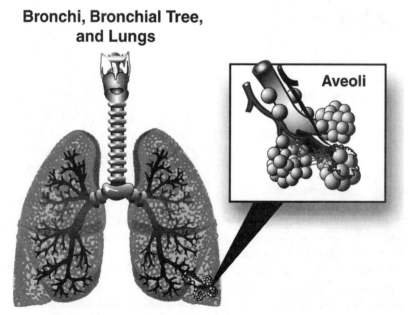

Figure 2–28. Larynx and lower respiratory passages. trachea, bronchi, lungs, terminal bronchioles and alveoli. From *Speech and Voice Science* (2nd ed.) by A. Behrman. Copyright © 2013 by Plural Publishing, Inc. Reprinted with permission.

Bronchioles/Bronchi

Function

These structures represent the main passageway for air into and out of the lungs. They are a conduit for airflow, so, like in the trachea, no gas exchange takes place here.

Structures and Spaces

There are two main-stem bronchi that extend off the trachea. The bronchi are similar in structure to the trachea but contain more smooth muscle fibers and are lined with psuedostratified, ciliated, columnar epithelium as well. Branches arise from these main bronchi called secondary bronchi. Further branching off the bronchi are bronchioles, which lead to the alveoli. The alveoli are sacs that occur in clusters at the terminal ends of the bronchioles, where the eventual exchange of oxygen (O_2) and carbon dioxide (CO_2) occurs.

> Clinical Note: *Asthma.* Asthma is caused by a swelling of the lining of the bronchi and bronchioles, as well as spasms of the smooth muscle of these passages. These swelling and muscle spasms cause wheezing and the sensation of shortness of breath. Asthma may be triggered by a variety of factors, including environmental allergens and illness. The prevalence of asthma in children continues to increase. As of 2009, the Centers for Disease Control and Prevention reported that 7.1 million children in the United States had asthma. As a voice clinician, you must understand that consistent use of inhalers with asthma medication (corticosteroids) has been associated with increased complaints of hoarseness (e.g., Gallivan, Gallivan, & Gallivan, 2007).

Lungs/Thoracic Cavity

Function

The purpose of the lungs is for gas exchange, that is, the delivery of oxygen to the bodily organs and the removal of carbon dioxide (CO_2).

Structures and Spaces

The lungs begin to develop at 4 weeks gestation but do not fully mature until just before birth. The lungs are contained within the thoracic cavity, the dimensions of which change through muscular contraction. The diaphragm is the main muscle of respiration and separates the thorax from the abdomen. Its contraction during inspiration pulls it downward, which in turn increases the vertical dimension of the thorax during inspiration. Additional expansion results from the contraction of the external intercostal muscles and other accessory muscles of inspiration, which elevate the rib cage. The lungs themselves consist of elastic tissue and are essentially passive structures during the speech breathing process. The lungs have a linkage to the diaphragm and the rib cage with a substance called pleura. This linkage allows the lungs to expand with the contraction of the inspiratory muscles.

Contained within the lungs at the terminal ends of the bronchioles are structures called alveoli, which are surrounded by capillaries (see Figure 2–28). At full term, a newborn has approximately 50 million alveoli. There is a rapid period of growth from birth to age 3 years during which this number will increase to 300 million (Parida, 2003). Here, oxygen from inhaled air enters the bloodstream and carbon dioxide leaves the blood and enters the lungs to be exhaled. This process of oxygen and carbon dioxide exchange is critical to human life. We will see later in this section that although speech breathing

Clinical Note: *Pulmonary surfactant.* Pulmonary surfactant is a substance that reduces the surface tension of the alveoli and prevents their collapse. Surfactant is not produced by pneumocyte cells in the lungs until 24 weeks gestation. Sufficient production is not observed until 35 weeks gestation. A medication called beta-methasone can be given to the pregnant mother to increase fetal surfactant production. Synthetic surfactant is administered to very premature infants at birth to aid lung function. Premature infants are susceptible to respiratory distress syndrome due to a lack of development of the respiratory system and may require oxygen support with or without mechanical ventilation.

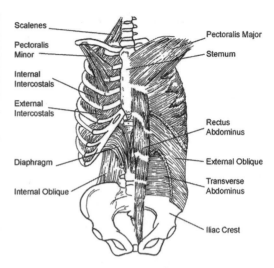

Figure 2–29. Diaphragm and accessory muscles of respiration. From *Voice Disorders* (2nd ed.) by C. Sapienza and B. Hoffman-Ruddy. Copyright © 2013 by Plural Publishing, Inc. Reprinted with permission.

Clinical Note: *Respiration vs. ventilation.* Respiration is the actual exchange of gases (O_2 and CO_2) that occurs in the lungs. Ventilation is a mechanical term referring to the process of moving air in and out of the lungs.

dimension of the lungs, thus increasing the volume. The contraction of the diaphragm occurs for all inspirations during rest and during activities such as speaking and singing. Another primary inspiratory muscle group is the external intercostals (Figure 2–30). The

alters resting breathing patterns, this alteration is generally not significant enough to disturb this important physiologic process.

Muscles of Respiration

Muscles of Inspiration

The primary muscle of inspiration is the diaphragm. This is a dome-shaped muscle that separates the thoracic and abdominal cavities (Figure 2–29). When the diaphragm contracts, it lowers, increasing the vertical

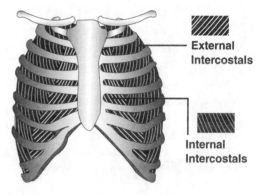

Figure 2–30. Rib cage and intercostal muscles. From *Speech and Voice Science* (2nd ed.) by A. Behrman. Copyright © 2013 by Plural Publishing, Inc. Reprinted with permission.

contraction of this muscle group serves to elevate the rib cage, increasing the horizontal dimension of the thoracic cavity. Accessory muscles of inspiration include muscles such as the sternocleidomastoid, pectoralis major, and pectoralis minor (see Figure 2–29). These muscles assist in inspiring larger volumes during speech, singing, and exercise.

Muscles of Expiration

Muscles that assist in active expiratory activities are located primarily in the abdominal and thoracic regions. These muscles primarily include the internal intercostals, rectus abdominus, external and internal obliques, and the transverse muscle (see Figure 2–29).

The Physiology of Breathing

The previous sections described the structural components of the respiratory system. In this section, the process of breathing incorporating all of the structural components will be discussed. The basic process of breathing involves moving air in and out of the respiratory system by increasing and decreasing the air pressure in the lungs.

Inhalation

During inspiration, the thoracic cavity is expanded, and subsequently the volume of the lungs increases. According to Boyle's law, there is an inverse relationship between volume and pressure when the temperature is kept constant. Therefore, when the volume of the lungs increases, the pressure in the lungs, more specifically the alveolar pressure, decreases (below atmospheric pressure). Air molecules tend to move to areas of lower pressure, and therefore air from the atmosphere rushes into the lungs.

The volume of the lungs is made larger by several muscle contractions, including a contraction of the diaphragm, which flattens and lowers. When the diaphragm contracts, there is an increase in the vertical dimension of the lungs due to the pleural linkage between the diaphragm and the lungs. The external intercostal muscles also contract, which in turn raises the rib cage. Again, due to the pleural linkage between the rib cage and the lungs, elevation of the rib cage expands the lungs horizontally and increases the volume.

Exhalation

During the process of exhalation, the volume of the lungs decreases and the pressure inside the lungs increases above atmospheric pressure. Thus, air molecules rush out to the area of lower pressure. The volume of the lungs is decreased by elastic recoil forces, which involves relaxation of the diaphragm and external intercostals.

The process of inhalation and exhalation described above represents breathing at rest or tidal breathing. During tidal breathing, the inspiratory and expiratory phases are of equal lengths. In adults, about 12 to 18 breaths per minute (bpm) typically occur at rest, while breaths per minute may be up to 30 to 60 in a newborn. Humans are able to breathe volumes much larger than those observed at rest. When an individual takes in the largest breath he possibly can, the volume from that breath is called *vital capacity* (VC). We are interested in the measurement of VC, as the amount of air inhaled prior to a speech utterance is typically described in a percentage of VC. During comfortable, conversational speech breathing, we generally inhale to about 60% of VC. If we are speaking very loudly or we want to produce a long singing segment, we may take in a larger breath (a higher percentage of VC) to be able to generate a larger amount of pressure from the lungs for vocal fold vibration.

During speech production, the inspiration generally encompasses 10% of the breathing cycle, whereas speech on expiration encompasses 90% of the cycle. The inspiratory muscles perform a quick, rapid contraction prior to the utterance to inhale the necessary volume for the intended utterance. The ability to quickly inspire in individuals who have healthy respiratory systems reduces the interruption of long pauses for phrasing. The inspiratory muscles are also utilized to control the rate of expiratory airflow during the expiratory phase of speech as well. This process is called inspiratory checking.

Speech breathing patterns noted in young children through and up to adolescence has been examined in the literature (Boliek, Hixon, Watson, & Morgan, 1996; Hoit et al., 1990; Stathopoulos & Sapienza, 1993). Generally, it has been observed that adultlike speech breathing patterns emerge prior to puberty. Children tend to breathe in larger lung volumes and terminate breaths at lower volumes than adults. Breathing efficiency (breathing in only needed volumes) appears to develop throughout childhood. There are several ways to measure respiratory function. For patients who have significant limitations to airflow or respiratory disease, the ability to interpret evaluations of their respiratory function will be important.

The Physiology of Phonation

In this last section of Chapter 2, we present the current understanding of the physiology of phonation, starting with basic concepts and terminology. Simply stated, phonation (or voicing) is caused by vocal fold vibration. The physiology of phonation refers to the mechanisms underlying the sound produced by TVF vibration. Normal, healthy phonation relies on the anatomy and physiology described in the preceding sections.

The Basics

Elements key to the physiology of phonation include those related to: (1) the position of the TVFs or shape of the glottis during various phonatory activities, (2) the muscular forces, including the length and tension of the TVFs, (3) condition of the vocal fold cover, (4) pressure and flow of pulmonary air up to and through the larynx, (5) interaction of that airflow with the soft tissue of the vocal fold cover, (6) behavior of the air stream in and around the glottis, and (7) the influence of the upper vocal tract on the sound generated.

The shape of the glottis is determined by the position of the TVFs. Recall that if the vocal folds are completely adducted, they are in the midline (closed) position. If they are abducted, the TVFs are apart from each other (open) to some degree (e.g., partial to narrow to wide separation). Adduction is accomplished with contraction of the lateral cricoarytenoid muscles, which rotate and rock the vocal process down and medially, and the transverse and oblique interarytenoids, which pull the arytenoids medially. When the TVFs are adducted, the arytenoids are closely approximated. Abduction is accomplished when there is contraction of the posterior cricoarytenoid muscles, which rotate and rock the vocal processes of the arytenoids back and out, moving the TVFs laterally.

The length and tension of the vocal folds change depending on the contraction of the intrinsic laryngeal muscles. Contraction of the thyroarytenoid (TA) muscles reduces the distance between the thyroid cartilage and arytenoids, thus shortening the length of the vocal folds, which in turn creates a thicker or more rounded vocal fold edge. In contrast, contraction of the cricothyroid (CT) muscle pulls or rocks the thyroid cartilage down and forward (toward the cricoid cartilage), thereby lengthening and thinning the TVFs as well as bringing an increase in tension to the medial edges.

Clinical Note: The larynx is considered a valve, and the degree of compression or lack thereof during closure will impact vocal quality and efficiency. For example, if the TVFs are too tightly approximated, elevated phonation threshold pressures will be needed to initiate phonation, and glottic airflow rates will be reduced. The resulting voice quality may be rough or pressed. If the TVFs are not sufficiently approximated, glottic airflow rates will increase and the voice quality will be breathy with less volume. Glottic configuration during a loud whisper is one in which the vocal folds are in a partially abducted position but with excess tension of the vocal fold edge.

As mentioned before, the health and pliability of the vocal fold cover are essential to normal vibratory behavior. The medial edges of the TVFs passively vibrate on the airstream as it passes through the glottis, so any abnormalities of the vocal fold cover (e.g., scarring, masses) can alter the rate or frequency of vibration, thus changing the sound/quality of the voice. Pulmonary airflow is the power source for phonation, so the control of pulmonary airflow is also critical to phonation. Although initiating and sustaining phonation do not require large volumes or high pressures of air, a consistent, well-regulated flow *is* needed. How this airflow interacts with the subglottic, glottic, supraglottic, and upper vocal tract to both impact vibration and give distinct qualities to the sound produced is of high importance to voice scientists and clinicians alike.

Theories of Phonation

Our current understanding of phonation is largely derived from the work of Van den Berg (1958), who described the myoelastic-aerodynamic theory of phonation. The basis of this theory states that vocal fold vibration involves muscular (myo) forces, the elasticity (elastic) of the vocal fold tissue, and intraglottic negative pressures created during airflow through a constricted glottal space. The suction forces resulting from these negative intraglottic pressures are attributed to the Bernoulli effect. These aerodynamic forces play a role in drawing the lower, then the upper lip of the medial vocal fold edge back to midline. Yet the original descriptions that largely focused on the Bernoulli effect were insufficient to explain the full role that aerodynamic forces play in initiating and sustaining phonation. Expansion of the myoelastic aerodynamic theory by Titze (1994) has advanced our understanding of the aerodynamics and self-sustaining aspects of vocal fold vibration. These later theories also took into consideration the cover-body structure of the vocal folds, including the inclusion of the two- and three-mass models (Story & Titze, 1995). Simply stated, the two-mass model refers to the action of the inferior and superior aspects of the vocal fold edge, whereas the three-mass model adds in the (action/influence) of the vocalis muscle during sustained vibration. The following is the sequence of aerodynamic and laryngeal events that occur when voice is produced. It is important to note that, to date, theories of phonation have not been described differently for children versus adults.

■ Phonation starts with the TVFs in a nearly or completely adducted position, permitting the buildup of subglottic air pressure.
■ The resistance of the soft, pliable vocal fold edge is overcome when sufficient subglottic *driving* pressure is reached (phonation threshold pressure), forcing apart first the lower, then the upper lip of the vocal fold edge.
■ As air flows through the glottis, the speed of the airflow increases through the constricted

glottal space (Bernoulli's law). The medial edges of the vocal folds are displaced in vertical and lateral dimensions.

■ This vertical and lateral tissue displacement initiates a mucosal (cover) wave motion across the surface of the vocal fold.

■ The Bernoulli effect and natural recoil of elastic forces within the vocal fold tissue draw back to midline first the lower, then the upper lip of the vocal fold edge.

■ Each cycle of vibration has an open phase (displacement as the intraglottal pressures are higher) and a closed phase (as the intraglottal pressure becomes negative), where there is a return to the medial (or near medial) approximation of the vocal fold.

■ The intraglottic space changes with the continuing changes of flow and pressure and with continued airflow and the action of the opening and closing of the glottis. This action will continue to repeat and in fact is repeated hundreds of times per second during sustained sound production (Titze, 1995).

■ Titze also describes the contribution of the supraglottic air column, where the air molecules of each cycle of the sound pressure wave (condensation and rarefaction) create a top-down loading effect that assists in sustaining phonation.

■ At the end of the phonatory segment, the TVFs will abduct by the action of the posterior cricoarytenoid muscle, the glottis is open, and regular respiration resumes.

In the description above, the airflow is upward, with *top-down* loading created by the supraglottal air column. In the past decade, however, a number of investigators studying fluid flow dynamics have sought to understand and determine the role that airflow separation and the rotational airflow in vortices (created by airflow through and above the glottis) play on the speed of vocal fold closure and resulting voice quality, particu-

Note: It is common for students to confuse the open and closed phases of a vibratory cycle with opening (abduction) and closing (adduction) of the glottis by action of the muscles and arytenoids. Remember that the TVFs remain in an adducted or nearly adducted position by the isotonic contraction of the intrinsic laryngeal muscles, and only the edges are blown open during vibration (Figures 2–31 and 2–32).

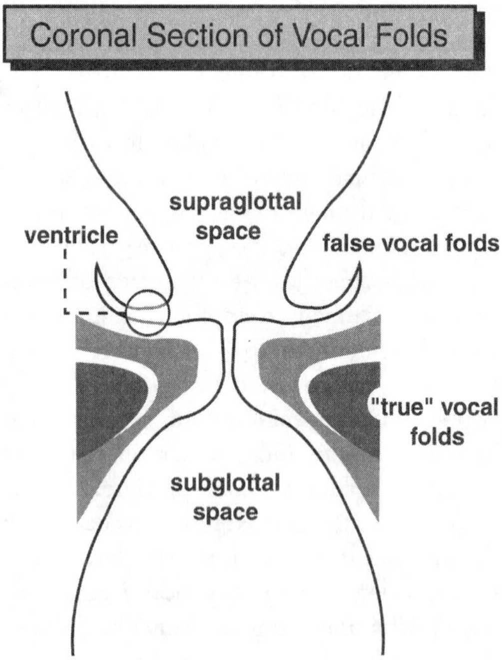

larly in terms of loudness and the production of high-frequency harmonics (Alipour & Scherer, 2000; Khosla, Murugappan & Gutmark, 2008; Khosla, Murugappan, Gutmark,

Figure 2–31. Schematic of a coronal view of a complete glottal cycle of vocal fold vibration. From *Speech and Voice Science* (2nd ed.) by A. Behrman. Copyright © 2013 by Plural Publishing, Inc. Reprinted with permission.

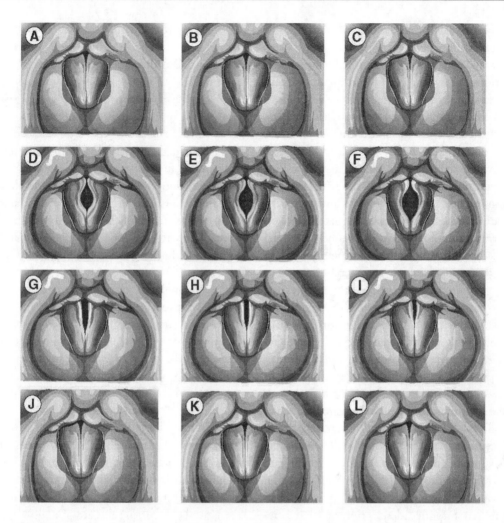

Figure 2–32. Schematic of a superior view of a glottal cycle of vocal fold vibration. **A** depicts the start of the vibratory cycle with the vocal folds in a near complete adducted position. Subsequent images (**B–L**) depict the onset of vibration through the full open and closed phase of the vibratory cycle. From *Speech and Voice Science* (2nd ed.) by A. Behrman. Copyright © 2013 by Plural Publishing, Inc. Reprinted with permission.

& Scherer, 2007; ; Titze, 2006). Using computational, computer, and animal modeling, these and similarly important investigations are adding to our knowledge about the aerodynamic principles underlying phonation. In time, a more sophisticated understanding of the aerodynamics of phonation will inform more sophisticated approaches to both surgical and behavioral clinical voice care.

Pitch and Intensity Changes

Pitch is the perceptual correlate of frequency and refers to how high or low a voice sounds. Frequency, or the number of cycles per second the vocal folds vibrate, is often measured in hertz (Hz) and is largely dependent on the interplay of the length, tension, and stiffness of the vocal fold body and cover (Kent, 1997) as controlled by the action of TA and CT muscles. In general, vibration of longer (thus larger) vocal folds results in a lower average fundamental frequency (as in an adult), and vibration of shorter vocal folds (as in a child) will result in higher average fundamental frequencies. Yet for any individual to increase frequency, there has to be a lengthening of the vocal folds, which will occur when there is muscular contraction of the CT. Contraction of the CT muscle stretches and tenses the vocal fold cover, thus reducing its mass. This permits the fold to vibrate at higher rates. Recall that the CT muscle pulls the thyroid cartilage down and forward, thereby lengthening the body of the vocal folds and decreasing the mass and increasing the tension of the cover. Increased vocal fold tension is a main component of increased frequency and requires higher subglottic pressures to initiate and sustain the higher rates of vibration. Lower frequencies are possible when there is increased mass and reduced tension of the vocal fold cover. This typically occurs when the TA muscle contracts and thus shortens the vocal folds, resulting in the cover of the folds becoming slack and rounded. The reader should be aware that these descriptions are a rather simplified description of what is really a dynamic muscle/tension/cover control relationship. Recall that the vocalis or medial portion of the TA muscle is considered a "tensor." The impact of vocalis tension on vocal fold vibration is influenced by discrete adjustments during active pitch change. The frequency range for human vocal folds is generally between 80 and 500 Hz during conversational speech and higher during infant cries and singing (Raphael, Borden, & Harris, 2007). Chapter 5 contains pediatric normative data for the frequency and aerodynamic values.

Intensity is the perceptual correlate of loudness and refers to how loud or soft a voice sounds. Average intensity (I_0), typically measured in decibels/sound pressure level (dB/SPL) refers to particle displacement during vibration and is dependent on the amplitude of vibration. To increase intensity, speakers use higher subglottic pressures to drive the vocal folds apart (amplitude of vibration), which results in a more rapid rate of closure. The greater degree of amplitude of vibration allows more air to rush through, resulting in the excitation of more air molecules and thus a greater acoustic energy. With the greater speed of closure and degree of amplitude of vibration, there is a more rapid cutoff and longer closed phase of the vibratory cycle (Behrman, 2013). Increase in F_0 also relies on increased subglottal pressures and increases in vocal fold tension. The relationship of increased intensity and higher pitch production is easily observed in the voices and cries of children.

Resonance

Resonance is a broad term used in the area of speech and voice that refers to the distinct frequencies associated with speech sounds or the "richness and timbre" of the voice. Resonance is a naturally occurring feature of a vibrating system and in voice and speech production and refers to the modification (intensification or damping) of the sound by the shape and configuration of the vocal tract. A resonator is something that is set into vibration (e.g., portions of the pharyngeal wall, nasopharynx, oral cavity) by another source of vibration (e.g., vocal folds). The "source filter theory" (Fant, 1960) of vowel production describes periodic vocal fold vibration as the source of sound that is modified or filtered by the length and configuration of the pharynx and oral cavity. Frequencies generated by the vocal folds are selectively filtered (for intensification or damping) within the vocal tract being influenced by the placement and action of the articulators. Therefore, resonance contributes extensively to the distinct sounds of speech and voice quality. Abnormalities of resonant qualities (e.g., hyper or hyponasality) are generally reserved for describing speech resulting from deviations in the valving action of the nasopharyngeal port. In Chapter 5 we discuss how we can measure intensity (dB/SPL), the average fundamental frequency (F^0) of a voice sample, its *harmonics* (multiples of F^0), and *formants* or resonances of the vocal tract. Behavioral manipulation of resonance, sometimes referred to as "focus," is also a common component of voice therapy. Sometimes described as a "subset" of voice production, it is important to realize that resonance relies on the interdependence of respiratory-vocal-articulatory processes.

Chapter Summary

In this chapter we have presented information fundamental to understanding voice production. Knowing the individual parts of the anatomy and respective physiology of the upper aerodigestive tract and pulmonary system is critical. Of greater importance is how the individual parts and regions function together for the production of human voice. This is critical to the clinician's ability to evaluate or treat any type of childhood voice disorder. You now know that voice changes dramatically from infancy to adulthood, due mainly to anatomic changes in the larynx that occur during development.

Important histological studies of the vocal folds have documented the microstructural changes in the vocal folds that occur over time. These observations help us understand how voice production changes during childhood. Moreover, it is necessary to consider the microstructural changes when planning care of pediatric voice. For example, the lack of layer structure in the lamina propria in young patients may require a novel surgical approach if in fact surgery is the best solution (Hartnick, Rehbar, & Prasad, 2005). Understanding the hormone regulation of vocal fold development may help us determine an appropriate timing for applying therapy or training techniques for adult voice. Vocal maturity is an important factor to consider when treating young performing voices. Many young singers are eager to sing adult repertoires, but singing repertoires that do not fit their voice can increase their risk of vocal injury.

Understanding the relationship between biological maturity of the vocal fold and vocal maturity and how biological maturity influences the risk of vocal fold injury is important. Whether mechanical stress from phonation contributes to the developmental changes in the lamina propria is an intriguing question, as it may influence the choice of voice therapy techniques. Another intriguing question may be how the biochemical difference between the pediatric and adult vocal folds influences healing process of the tissue. More information on the microstructure of the vocal fold and its relationship to vocal fold pathology and treatment is presented in later chapters.

References

Alberts, B., Johnson, A., Lewis, J., Raff, M., Roberts, K., & Walter, P. (2002). Extracellular matrix of animals. *Molecular biology of the cell* (4th ed.). New York, NY: Garland Science. http://www.ncbi.nlm.nih.gov/books /NBK26810.

Alipour, F., & Scherer, R. C. (2004). Flow separation in a computational oscillating vocal fold model. *Journal of the Acoustical Society of America, 116*(3), 1710–1719.

Allen, K. (2012). Gastro-oesophageal reflux in children. What's the worry? *Australian Family Physician, 41*(5), 268–272.

Behrman, A. (2013). *Speech and voice science* (2nd ed.). San Diego, CA: Plural Publishing.

Bluestone, C. D., Stool, S. E., Alper, C. M., Arjmand, E. M., Casselbrant, M. L., Dohar, J. E., & Yellon, R. F. (2003). *Pediatric otolaryngology, volume 1* (4th ed.). Philadelphia, PA: Saunders.

Boliek, C., Hixon, T., Watson, P., & Morgan, W. (1996). Vocalization and breathing during the first year of life. *Journal of Voice, 10*(1), 1–22.

Buhler, R. B., Sennes, L. U., Mauad, T., Melo, E. C., Silva, L. F., & Saldiva, P. H. (2008). Collagen fiber and versican distribution within the lamina propria of fetal vocal folds. *Laryngoscope, 118*(2), 371–374. doi: 10.1097/MLG.0b013e318159aa0d.

Campanozzi, A., Boccia, G., Pensabene, L., Panetta, F., Marseglia, A., Strisciuglio, P., . . . Staiano, A. (2009). Prevalence and natural history of gastroesophageal reflux: Pediatric prospective study. *Pediatrics, 123*, 779–783.

Catten, M., Gray, S. D., Hammond, T. H., Zhou, R., & Hammond, E. (1998). Analysis of cellular location and concentration in vocal fold lamina propria. *Otolaryngology-Head and Neck Surgery, 118*(5), 663–667.

Fant, G. (1960). *Acoustic theory of speech production.* The Hague: Mouton.

Gallivan, G. J., Gallivan, K. H., & Gallivan, H. K. (2007). Inhaled corticosteroids: Hazardous effects on voice. An update. *Journal of Voice, 21*(1), 101–111.

Gray, S. D. (2000). Cellular physiology of the vocal folds. *Otolaryngology Clinics of North America, 33*(4), 679–698.

Gray, S. D., Titze, I. R., Chan, R., & Hammond, T. H. (1999). Vocal fold proteoglycans and their influence on biomechanics. *Laryngoscope, 109*(6), 845–854.

Hammond, T. H., Gray, S. D., Butler, J., Zhou, R., & Hammond, E. (1998). Age- and gender-related elastin distribution changes in human vocal folds. *Otolaryngology-Head and Neck Surgery, 119*(4), 314–322.

Hartnick, C. J., & Bosley, M. E. (2008). *Pediatric voice disorders.* San Diego, CA: Plural Publishing.

Hartnick, C. J., Rehbar, R., & Prasad, V. (2005). Development and maturation of the pediatric human vocal fold lamina propria. *Laryngoscope, 115*(1), 4–15. doi: 0.1097/01.mlg.0000150685.54893.e9.

Hemler, R. J., Wieneke, G. H., & Dejonckere, P. H. (1997). The effect of relative humidity of inhaled air on acoustic parameters of voice in normal subjects. *Journal of Voice, 11*(3), 295–300.

Hemler, R. J., Wieneke, G. H., Lebacq, J., & Dejonckere, P. H. (2001). Laryngeal mucosa elasticity and viscosity in high and low relative air humidity. *European Archives of Otorhinolaryngology, 258*(3), 125–129.

Hirano, M. (1977). Structure and vibratory behavior of the vocal folds. In M. Sawashima & F. S. Cooper (Eds.), *Dynamic aspects of speech production* (pp. 13–27). Tokyo: University of Tokyo Press.

Hirano, M. (1981). *Clinical examination of voice.* Vienna/New York: Springer-Verlag.

Hirano, M., Kurita, S., & Nakashima, T. (1983). Growth, development, and aging of human vocal folds. In D. Bless & J. Abbs (Eds.), *Vocal fold physiology* (pp. 23–43). San Diego, CA: College-Hill Press.

Hirano, M., Kurita, S., & Sakaguchi, S. (1989). Ageing of the vibratory tissue of human vocal folds. Acta Oto-Laryngologica, 107(5–6), 428–433.

Hoit, J., Hixon, T., Watson, P., & Morgan, W. (1990). Speech breathing in children and adolescents. *Journal of Speech and Hearing Research, 33*, 51–69.

Hollien, H. (2012). On pubescent voice change in males. *Journal of Voice, 26*(2), e29.

Hollien, H., & Shipp, T. (1972). Speaking fundamental frequency and chronologic age in males. *Journal of Speech and Hearing Research, 15*(1), 155–159.

Kent, R. D. (1997). *The speech sciences.* San Diego, CA: Singular Publishing Group.

Khosla, S., Murugappan, S., & Gutmark, E. (2008). What can vortices tell us about vocal fold vibration and voice production? *Current Opinions in Otolaryngology-Head and Neck Surgery, 16*, 183–187.

Khosla, S., Murugappan, S., Gutmark, E., & Scherer, R. (2007). Vortical flow field during phonation in an excised canine larynx model. *Annals of Otology, Rhinology and Laryngology, 116*(3), 217–228.

Larsen, W. J. (1993). *Human embryology.* New York, NY: Churchill Livingstone.

Leydon, C., Sivasankar, M., Falciglia, D. L., Atkins, C., & Fisher, K. V. (2009). Vocal fold surface hydration: A review. *Journal of Voice, 23*(6), 658–665. doi: 10.1016/j.jvoice .2008.03.010

Madruga de Melo, E. C., Lemos, M., Aragao Ximenes Filho, J., Sennes, L. U., Nascimento Saldiva, P. H., & Tsuji, D. H. (2003). Distribution of collagen in the lamina propria of the human vocal fold. *Laryngoscope, 113* (12), 2187–2191. doi: 10.1097/00005537-200312000-00027

Mescher, A. (2010). *Junqueira's basic histology: Text and atlas* (12th ed.). New York, NY: McGraw-Hill Medical.

Miller, J. L. (2003). Emergence of oropharyngeal, laryngeal and swallowing activity in the developing fetal upper aerodigestive tract: An ultrasound evaluation. *Early Human Development, 71*(1), 61–87.

Moore, K. L. (1992). *Clinically oriented anatomy* (3rd ed.). Baltimore, MD: Williams & Wilkins.

Moore, P., & von Leden, H. (1961). The mechanics of the cricoarytenoid joint. *Archives of Otolaryngology, 73*, 541–550.

Murray, T., & Carrau, R. L. (2006). *Clinical management of swallowing disorders* (2nd ed.). San Diego, CA: Plural Publishing.

Myer, C. M., Cotton, R. T., & Schott, S. R. (1995). *Pediatric airway: An interdisciplinary approach.* Philadelphia, PA: J. B. Lippincott.

Nacci, A., Fattori, B., Basolo, F., Filice, M. E., De Jeso, K., Giovannini, L., & Ursino, F. (2011). Sex hormone receptors in vocal fold tissue: A theory about the influence of sex hormones in the larynx. *Folia Phoniatrica and Logopeadicas, 63*(2), 77–82. doi: 10.1159/000316136

Newman, S. R., Butler, J., Hammond, E. H., & Gray, S. D. (2000). Preliminary report on hormone receptors in the human vocal fold. *Journal of Voice, 14*(1), 72–81.

Nita, L. M., Battlehner, C. N., Ferreira, M. A., Imamura, R., Sennes, L. U., Caldini, E. G., & Tsuji, D. H. (2009). The presence of a vocal ligament in fetuses: A histochemical and ultrastructural study. *Journal of Anatomy, 215*(6), 692–697. doi: 10.1111/j.1469-7580 .2009.01146.x

Parida, S. K. (2003). Respiratory disorders of the newborn. In C. Bluestone, S. Stool, C. Alper, E. Arjmand, L. Casselbrant, J. Dohar, & R. Yellon (Eds.), *Pediatric otolaryngology* (2nd ed.). Philadelphia, PA: Saunders.

Prades, J. M., Dumollard, J. M., Duband, S., Timoshenko, A., Richard, C., Dubois, M. D., . . . Peoc'h, M. (2010). Lamina propria of the human vocal fold: Histomorphometric study of collagen fibers. *Surgical Radiological Anatomy, 32*(4), 377–382. doi: 10.1007/s00276-009-0577-9

Raphael, L. J., Borden, G. J., & Harris, K. S. (2007). *Speech science primer* (5th ed.). Baltimore, MD: Lippincott Williams & Wilkins.

Rosenberg, T. L., & Schweinfurth, J. M. (2009). Cell density of the lamina propria of neonatal vocal folds. *Annals of Otology, Rhinology and Laryngology, 118*(2), 87–90.

Sapienza, C., & Hoffman-Ruddy, B. (2009). *Voice disorders.* San Diego, CA: Plural Publishing.

Sato, K., & Hirano, M. (1997). Age-related changes of elastic fibers in the superficial layer of the lamina propria of vocal folds. *Annals of Otology, Rhinology and Laryngology, 106*(1), 44–48.

Sato, K., Hirano, M., & Nakashima, T. (2001). Fine structure of the human newborn and infant vocal fold mucosae. *Annals of Otology Rhinology and Laryngology, 110*(5 Pt. 1), 417–424.

Schneider, B., Cohen, E., Stani, J., Kolbus, A., Rudas, M., Horvat, R., & van Trotsenburg, M. (2007). Towards the expression of sex hormone receptors in the human vocal fold. *Journal of Voice, 21*(4), 502–507. doi: 10.1016/j .jvoice.2006.01.002

Schweinfurth, J. M., & Thibeault, S. L. (2008). Does hyaluronic acid distribution in the larynx relate to the newborn's capacity for crying? *Laryngoscope, 118*(9), 1692–1699. doi: 10.1097/MLG.0b013e3181782754

Stathopoulos, E., & Sapienza, C. (1993). Respiratory and laryngeal measures of children during vocal intensity variation. *Journal of the Acoustical Society of America, 94*, 2531–2543.

Stemple, J. C., Glaze, L. E., & Klaben, B. G. (2000). *Clinical voice pathology: Theory and management* (3rd ed.). San Diego, CA: Singular Publication Group.

Story, B. H., & Titze, I. R. (1995). Voice simulation with the body-cover model of the vocal folds. *Journal of the Acoustical Society of America, 97*(2), 1249–1260.

Thibeault, S. L., Gray, S. D., Bless, D. M., Chan, R. W., & Ford, C. N. (2002). Histologic and rheologic characterization of vocal fold scarring. *Journal of Voice, 16*(1), 96–104.

Titze, I. R. (1994). *Principles of voice production.* Upper Saddle River, NJ: Prentice-Hall.

Titze, I. R. (2006). Theoretical analysis of maximum flow declination rate versus maximum area declination rate in phonation. *Journal of Speech-Language-Hearing Research, 49*(2): 439–447.

Van den Berg, J. W., (1958). Myo-elastic theory of voice production. *Journal of Speech and Hearing Research, 1*, 227–244.

Voelter, C., Kleinsasser, N., Joa, P., Nowack, I., Martinez, R., Hagen, R., & Voelker, H. U. (2008). Detection of hormone receptors in the human vocal fold. *European Archives of Otorhinolaryngology, 265*(10), 1239–1244. doi: 10.1007/s00405-008-0632-x

Ward, P. D., Thibeault, S. L., & Gray, S. D. (2002). Hyaluronic acid: Its role in voice. *Journal of Voice, 16*(3), 303–309.

Ximenes Filho, J. A., Tsuji, D. H., do Nascimento, P. H., & Sennes, L. U. (2003). Histologic changes in human vocal folds correlated with aging: A histomorphometric study. *Annals of Otology, Rhinology and Laryngology, 112*(10), 894–898.

CHAPTER 3

Neural Controls of Voice

In this chapter we provide an overview of the central and peripheral nervous system controls needed to support the development and production of normal voice. Much of what we know about the neural controls of voicing come from animal-based research, since animal and mammalian species (e.g., songbirds, bats, whales) possess similar vegetative and (some) skilled vocalizations for communication. However, only humans possess the full continuum of phonatory functions that range from reflexive and protective laryngeal actions (e.g., cough) to the volitionally controlled and coordinated, highly skilled vocal movements needed to support speech. In children, the development of these precisely coordinated respiratory, phonatory, and articulatory actions occur in conjunction with the development of cognitive and linguistic skills, all of which are necessary requirements for vocalization-based communication abilities.

Use of imaging to examine cortical structures, pathways, and activity related to vocal motor control in normal and disordered adults is providing new insights into these important mechanisms. Functional magnetic resonance imaging (fMRI), transcranial magnetic stimulation (TMS), and various electro-physiologic measures (e.g., electromyography, or EMG) permit investigators to affirm, expand, or revise our knowledge related to established pathways and the impact of damage or disruption on their function. Expanding use of these techniques to study children presents obvious challenges, although an increasing number of brain imaging studies in children to examine the cortical controls of speech and language are being conducted (Szaflarski et al., 2012).

Vocalization and the Infant Cry

Most healthy human babies start life with a vigorous, loud cry. Albeit a reflexive act and one that follows the first real inhalation, the newborns' cry, their first use of voice, not only activates the respiratory system, but also signals health and communicates their arrival in the world. The sound of the cry, like all phonation, is generated by vibrations of the vocal folds within the larynx, powered by air expired from the lungs, shaped by the vocal tract, and accompanied by facial and extremity motor movements, all of which are ultimately controlled or influenced by multiple levels of the nervous system. The subsequent development of vocalization for purposes of communication requires an exquisite series of neurodevelopmental activities that start from the instant the newborn begins interacting with his or her environment. In the first weeks of life, infant cries quickly differentiate, indicating needs related to hunger, comfort, unhappiness, illness, and fatigue (Krueger, 1970). Extensive literature exists on the acoustic and respiratory features of various cries and how they change as the infant grows and develops. Importantly, from birth on, abnormal cries and vocalizations can signal congenital or acquired health conditions, serious acute illness, and developmental concerns (Hirschberg, Szende, Koltai & Illényi, 2009).

Various investigators have used different terminology to describe cry characteristics. These descriptions are based on acoustic features, as well as perceptual judgments, and have been studied for decades (Hirschberg et al., 2009). Categories of cry can include, "1. basic cry: simple expressive phonation; 2. turbulence cry: dysphonic cry characterized by excessive constriction of the upper airway; and 3. shift cry or hyperphonation where there is extremely high pitched components" (Hirschberg et al., 2009, p. 10). These categories have been used by others to assist in the further acoustic and perceptual differentiation of pathological cries.

Key acoustic parameters currently used to characterize cry include measures of average fundamental frequency (F_0) and formants, as well as duration of cry segments and melodic or pitch contour. The reported F_0 of most healthy cries (in infants) is around 450 Hz, though it can range between 400 and 600 Hz. The contour of cry also matters. For example, healthy cries tend to have rising and falling patterns, whereas pathologic cries tend to be more vacillating (fluctuating). Depending on the context, it is common to interpret the various patterns and force of cries

as the infant *indicating* a specific need, so how a parent or caregiver *perceives* and then reacts to a child's cry is also an important consideration. As the infant's cry signals a need, the ability of the parent to appropriately respond influences care and shapes early behavioral communicative interactions (Hirschberg et al., 2009).

> Clinical Note: At birth, a weak and high-pitched cry can signal the presence of a glottic web. A glottic web is the result of an incomplete separation of the vocal folds during embryogenesis. Stridor, or noisy inhalation during cry or feeding, can signal laryngomalacia. This is a condition whereby the cartilages of the larynx are extremely soft and prolapse into the laryngeal inlet during forced inhalation (Myer, Cotton, & Schott, 1995).

The different categories of non-cry infant vocalizations (e.g., coo, raspberries, squeals) can be observed during vocal play when the child does or does not have an audience. This vocal play is an important activity that permits the child the opportunity to explore and learn to exert control over his or her vocal behaviors. Vocal play occurs when the child is alone and as part of an early communicative exchange. Ultimately the sounds produced will be shaped into meaningful communication units and increase in response to reinforcement given by the mother or caregiver. Reinforcement from a caregiver can be in the form of exact imitation, eye contact and facial expression, and holding or something similarly socially rewarding (Palaez,

Virues-Ortega, & Gewirtz, 2011). The nature and frequency of reinforcement are important factors in establishing these essential prelinguistic vocal exchanges. The flexibility of infant vocalizations is uniquely human, and these are the phonatory precursors to speech. Children must also have intact auditory (and other sensory feedback) systems in order for them to develop truly sophisticated control over vocalization (Russo, Larson, & Kraus, 2008).

Another key consideration in the development of vocal motor control for non-cry vocalization is how it unfolds in conjunction with the development of other motor skills, particularly upper extremity (UE) motion (Oller, 2010). The development of the intentional control of vocalization has been described by some as having a direct relationship with the emergence of early skilled and rhythmic UE motions. Early canonical babbling is often accompanied by rhythmic motion of the arms (Iverson, 2010). The sequential development of controlled vocalizations and the timing of their control relative to other large motor extremity function have been extensively studied by Oller (2010). The relationship of (skilled) extremity movement and vocal development to the development of sophisticated language is a topic of some debate. There is the view that the speech sounds needed for language development are unique and innately available to the infant from birth. Alternatively, others view the development of skilled phonation and articulation as requiring input, practice, and coordination of these systems to occur in conjunction with the skilled movements of other systems. Close attention and careful study has been conducted on how the emergence and mastery of skilled extremity movement precedes that of speech. Each of these perspectives is important and readers are directed to the works of Iverson et al. to further their understanding.

Central Neural Controls

Vocal motor behavior involves respiratory, laryngeal, and supralaryngeal vocal tract mechanisms and can be globally described as being either reactive (innate) or learned. All levels of the nervous system are involved in voice production. Organization of the central nervous system (brain and spinal cord) involves hierarchical, lateral, and functional systems. *Hierarchical* refers to the levels of function (e.g., lower, or reflexive, to higher, or executive); *laterality* refers to the crossover of cortical and ascending/descending pathways from one side to the other; and *functional organization* refers to regions of the brain dedicated to certain functions (e.g., speech and language, vision, hearing) or locations (cortical, subcortical, etc.) (Luria, 1973).

Executive function associated with cognition, intelligence, language, planning and sequencing of motor movements, primary sensory perception, and secondary sensory integration are controlled at the highest cortical levels. Circuitry and systems influencing and refining motor movement, emotion, sensory integration, and so forth are generally located in the subcortical locations, such as the basal ganglia, limbic system, and cerebellum. Reflexive actions occur in the neural circuitry of the brainstem and spinal cord depending on where the stimulus is generated (e.g., extremities versus head and neck). Of course there are complex continuous and coordinated communications between lower and higher centers for all sensory motor function, including voicing.

Brainstem

Examination of the neural circuitry subserving vocal motor control has been conducted, in part, using animal studies. Delineation and differentiation of vocal function, as evident in animal versus mammalian (human and nonhuman) species, is important to note and is elegantly reviewed in work done by Jürgens (2002, 2009). In mammals, the brainstem contains multiple sites of sensory and motor neuron pools that interact with each other, as well as adjacent centers. These centers are dedicated to generating the life-sustaining neural activity necessary to the integration of respiratory, articulatory, vocal, and swallowing functions. Depending on the activity (function), these centers direct sensory signals coming in from the periphery to the appropriate motor neuron circuits. These circuits regulate basic primitive and protective (reflexive) responses, as well as more complicated and integrated responses (e.g., gagging versus chewing and swallowing) that require extensive networks of premotor neurons, motor neurons, and interneurons.

The primary centers for the integration of laryngeal, swallowing, and respiratory functions are located in the medulla. These centers are networks of neural circuits known as pattern generators (Miller, 1999). There are central pattern generators instrumental for the initiation and progression of the swallowing response; licking and chewing activity; and vocalization and respiration. Sensory information comes in from the larynx, pharynx, and respiratory centers via first-order sensory neurons to the nucleus tractus solitarius (NTS). The NTS is the major medullary sensory input center that receives information from the pharynx, larynx, and lungs and routes it to the premotor and motor neuron circuitry of the medulla as well as higher centers. Other sensation from the articulators and tongue are transmitted via the trigeminal and hypoglossal nerves to the spinal trigeminal tract and the NTS. In the case of reflexive type laryngeal responses (e.g.,

cough, laryngeal adductor response), information travels from the NTS to the nucleus ambiguous (NA) and dorsal motor nucleus of cranial nerve (CN) X. This region contains the premotor neurons and motor neurons for all of the intrinsic muscles of the larynx. For coordinated, sequential, and integrated vocal function, the relay of information involves multiple centers at all levels of the brainstem.

The area of the periaqueductal gray (PAG) of the midbrain is especially critical to the generation (initiation), intensity, and timing of laryngeal muscles during phonation. Animal and mammal studies (nonhuman and human) have revealed that electrical stimulation of this region will result in reactive or preprogrammed-type vocalizations (Jürgens, 2009). For example, depending on the animal and precise circuitry (within the PAG) hissing, meows, screaming, and certain types of cries can be elicited with electrical or chemical stimulation. In humans, stimulation of this region can produce similar vocalizations and even some laughter. Jürgens (2002) notes that in certain animals, destruction of this region will not change the acoustic characteristics of a vocal call but may eliminate it entirely, whereas interruption of lower medullary centers can result in significant alterations of acoustic features and rhythms. The circuits of the PAG communicate with the NA, but not by direct connections. Input to the PAG is by way of higher cortical and subcortical centers as well as from the inter- and premotor neurons received by the NTS below (Larson, 1988). As such, the PAG acts as a vocal relay center, influencing the basic phonatory processing (versus coordinating) function of vocal motor responses. Destruction of the PAG has been shown to result in mutism for both animals and humans (Jürgens, 2009).

Areas of the parabrachial nuclei in the pons also have neurons that are active during phonation, particularly for the integration of laryngeal respiratory function. As an integral part of the vocal motor pathway in mammals, this region is known to receive sensory input from the lungs and information regarding the movement of laryngeal cartilages, vocal fold tension, and subglottic pressure (Smotherman, Kobayasi, Ma, Zhang, & Metzner, 2006). Within the pontine-medullary brainstem, the reticular formation (RF) plays an important role in coordinating the patterning of acoustic features of vocal responses, as well as integrating respiratory, phonatory, and articulatory activity. In some species, destruction of the RF has resulted in severe alteration of the acoustic features of phonatory segments (Jürgens, 2009).

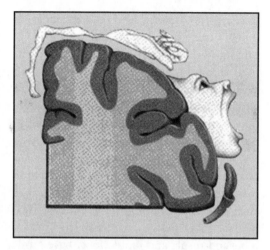

Figure 3–1. Coronal view of the homunculus (somatosensory and motor) cortex. From *Brain-Based Communication Disorders* by L. LaPointe. Copyright © 2010 by Plural Publishing, Inc. Reprinted with permission.

Cortical and Subcortical Controls

The precise central nervous system (CNS) controls and circuitry involved in voicing for fine motor control of intentional, learned, and even emotionally based communication are complex, and a full understanding of the exact mechanisms are still emerging. Multiple cortical regions are involved with more complex learned vocal behavior. It is well known that the motor strip of the cortex is topically mapped for all of the body's skilled motor movements. The lateral, lower (inferior) portions of the presylvian fissure are bilaterally mapped for the larynx and are referred to as the laryngeal motor cortex. The laryngeal motor cortex is inferior to areas of the mouth and face (Figure 3–1). In humans, these areas receive input from the premotor and supplementary motor cortex, where the planning and sequencing of patterned vocalization and speech are initiated and executed. This is also adjacent to Broca's area, the third inferior frontal convolution of the (left) frontal cortex, essential for the production of spoken language. These are the critical cortical regions

for the volitional, skilled control of speech, voice, and respiration. Of course, in order to learn, plan, sequence, and execute commands for vocalization and speech, the frontal (motor) cortex has to receive integrated sensory and linguistic information from the auditory cortex and parietal lobe. Depending on the exact site and extent of injury, and whether there is unilateral or bilateral involvement, diminished or complete loss of the ability to execute and fluently sequence voluntary vocalizations can occur.

Lateral dominance for the discrete control of skilled voice and speech movement is well described in the literature (Kingsley, 2000; Loucks, Poletto, Simonyan, Reynolds, & Ludlow, 2007; Ludlow, 2004; Luria, 1973; Simonyan, Ostuni, Ludlow, & Horowitz, 2009). The origins of left cerebral dominance for vocal and eventually linguistic function involve an understanding of the various evolutionary timelines offered in the literature. According to some studies, the development of the predominance of right-handedness is thought to be linked to the emergence of vocalizations during the period of primitive gestural communication (Corballis, 2003). For gross functional purposes, cortical representation of the larynx is thought to be bilateral (albeit somewhat unequal), similar to the upper face. Additional cortical and subcortical regions also play important roles in various aspects of voluntary controlled phonation for speech or speech-related activity. Multiple cortical areas, including the auditory cortex, parietal lobe, motor regions of the frontal lobe, and insula and limbic lobe, have a role in emotional and learned vocalizations (Poletto, Verdun, Strominger, & Ludlow, 2004). In functional imaging studies, activation of the anterior cingulate gyrus is observed for innate vocal tasks associated with emotion or the anticipation of emotional responses (Jürgens, 2002). For these types of vocal motor activities, projections from the motor cortex travel to lower brainstem centers by way of the pyramidal pathways, but not before being influenced by two important subcortical motor loops or circuits.

> The cingulate gyrus is part of the limbic system and is located deep to the frontal and parietal lobes just above and somewhat encircling the corpus callosum (Figure 3–2 shows the position of the corpus callosum).

The purpose of these two main motor loops is to refine, smooth, and balance motor movements required to accomplish specific skilled motor tasks. One loop involves the inhibitory and excitatory circuits of the basal ganglia, which influence the motor signal for skilled (in this case laryngeal) movements, before traveling down the pyramidal pathways to the medulla and cranial nerve nuclei.

> A depletion of the nigrostriatal dopaminergic neurons in this region (as in Parkinson disease [PD] and, in rare cases, pediatric onset of PD) and resulting alteration of *excitatory* influences may result in a reduction of the speed and precision of vocal motor control (or hypophonia) and articulation. With altered *inhibitory* controls, there can be an increase in activity of the excitatory circuitry, resulting in uncontrolled vocal motor activity, such as tics, tremors, or coughing. In children, congenital or acquired neurologic conditions or certain medication therapies can impact the integrity of these circuits, causing temporary, permanent, or a late onset of symptoms.

The second loop involves neural (motor) impulses that travel via connections between the the motor strip and the cerebellum and return to the motor strip of the cortex by way of the thalamus, before descending the pyramidal pathway to the brainstem. The influence of this circuit involves aspects of voice onset, regulation of fundamental frequency, precision, and coordination with other systems, including respiration. Cerebellar lesions, depending on their location and extent, will result in an incoordination of those elements of voice and speech.

There are two main vocal control pathways. One is uniquely human and is considered "direct," routing the "influenced motor signals" (as described above) directly from the areas of the cortex involved in intentional phonation (as described above) to the RF and premotor neurons of the cranial nerve nuclei in the medulla. If some of the "influencing" circuits (e.g., cerebellum or basal ganglia) are damaged, there can be movement of the vocal folds, but the timing and coordination of

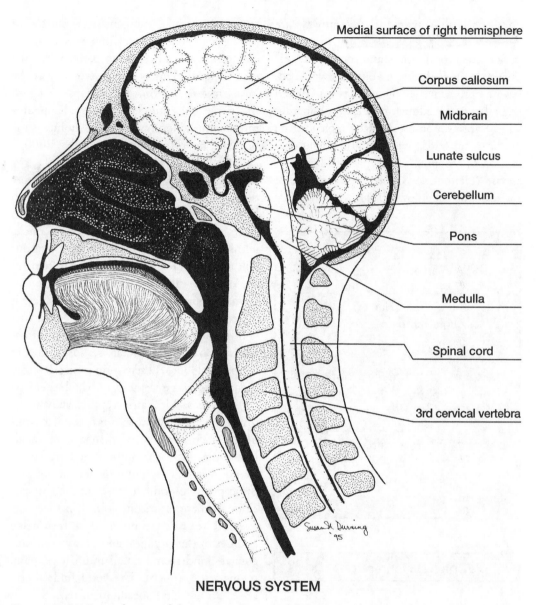

Medial surface of right hemisphere

Corpus callosum

Midbrain

Lunate sulcus

Cerebellum

Pons

Medulla

Spinal cord

3rd cervical vertebra

NERVOUS SYSTEM

Figure 3–2. Sagittal view of the main structures of the central nervous system. From *Anatomy and Physiology Study Guide for Speech and Hearing, Second Edition* by W. Culbertson, S. Christensen and D. Tanner. Copyright © 2013 by Plural Publishing, Inc. Reprinted with permission.

their use will be affected. The second loop is considered indirect and involves impulses from the limbic lobe to the PAG and then to the RF and laryngeal motor neurons in the medulla for vocal production readiness and innate vocalizations (Jürgens, 2009). In humans, if there is bilateral involvement of key cortical structures that control voluntary vocalization but the lower areas of the upper brainstem including the PAG are intact, innate vocalization is still possible (e.g., moaning, some cries).

In a healthy system, these pathways are constantly working in synchrony to accomplish needed vocalizations and vocal behaviors. For example, if during a voluntary vocal behavior a protective laryngeal reflex is triggered (e.g., laryngeal adductor reflex), phonation will be abruptly interrupted by rapid closure of the vocal folds. Interestingly, a volitional swallow can suppress the laryngeal adductor response (Henriquez, Schulz, Bielamowicz, & Ludlow, 2007; Ludlow, 2011).

> Clinical Note: Clinicians may work with their patients to attempt to alter the interaction of the voluntary and more automatic (reflexive) pathways. For example, chronic throat clearing could be a pattern of hyperreactive vocal behavior that is habituated over time. Even if the original stimulus is resolved, the throat clearing can continue. A common therapeutic strategy is to replace the throat clearing with a voluntary hard swallow in order to break the cycle and substitute a behavior that is not traumatizing to the vocal fold tissue.

Peripheral Neural Controls

Cranial Nerves

The peripheral nervous system includes the cranial and spinal nerves and the autonomic (sympathetic and parasympathetic) nervous system. Cranial nerves of the head and neck transmit (and regulate) sensory motor information to and from the CNS. Cranial nerves carrying motor information to muscles of the head and neck have their nuclei within the medulla of the brainstem. The nerve axons travel out to the end organs (e.g., muscles of the larynx, pharynx, and upper esophagus), acting as the final common pathway for the motor signal. This is also referred to as the lower motor neuron. The synapse between the nerve and muscle is called the neuromuscular junction, where acetylcholine is the principal neurotransmitter (Kingsley, 2000).

Cranial nerves carrying sensory information into the CNS from the larynx typically do so in a chain of three, the first of which have their nuclei in peripheral ganglion with fibers that synapse on second-order nuclei within the brainstem. Second-order neurons will typically cross over in the brainstem (to the opposite side of entrance) and carry information up to the thalamus, where there is a second synapse with the third neuron that will be the pathway for the sensory information to travel to the primary sensory cortex of the parietal lobe. All sensation is first detected by nerve ending receptors, of which there are several types. Mechanoreceptors activate by displacement; chemoreceptors respond to stimulants, such as water, salts, sugars, and acids (Rudolph, 1995, p. 329); stretch receptors found in muscles respond to elongation; proprioceptors respond to mechanical and positional changes within joints; nociceptors respond to pain stimulus; and free nerve endings of the laryngeal and pharyngeal mucosa respond to multiple stimuli (e.g., pain, temperature, touch). The vocal folds themselves do not have specific pain receptors, as noted by their ability to withstand constant vibration.

Cranial Nerve X—Vagus

The larynx and much of the pharynx and upper esophagus are innervated by the tenth cranial nerve, or CN X, the vagus nerve. It is the longest and most complex of the cranial nerves and descends deep into the thorax and abdomen. It is important to remember that it is a "mixed" nerve and thus relays both sensory and motor signals. The main trunks of the right and left vagus nerves exit the brainstem and then the skull via the jugular foramen and descend in the neck (on each side) between the jugular vein and carotid artery (Figure 3–3). Multiple branches leave the main trunk of the vagus, including the pharyngeal branch, the superior laryngeal branches (internal and external), and the recurrent laryngeal nerve. Motor innervation to the velum and pharyngeal constrictors is by way of the pharyngeal branch. Sensation from this region is by way of both CNs IX and X. These two nerves, along with fibers from CN XI, make up the pharyngeal plexus. Sensation from the supraglottic larynx (above the vocal folds) travels by way of the internal branch of the superior laryngeal nerve

(SLNib), while contraction of the cricothyroid muscle is accomplished by the external branch (SLNeb). The remainder of the intrinsic muscles of the larynx, the upper esophagus, and sensation from the trachea receive motor innervation by the recurrent laryngeal nerves (RLNs) and their branches (Figure 3–4). Importantly, the left and right RLNs follow different courses as they travel in the chest. This anatomic arrangement has important clinical implications (see box below). The right RLN branches from the main trunk and descends into the thorax to the level of the right subclavian artery, where it passes beneath and ascends up (and under the thyroid gland) to the larynx. The left RLN descends deeper into the thorax to the level of the aorta before passing underneath and ascending to the left side of the larynx.

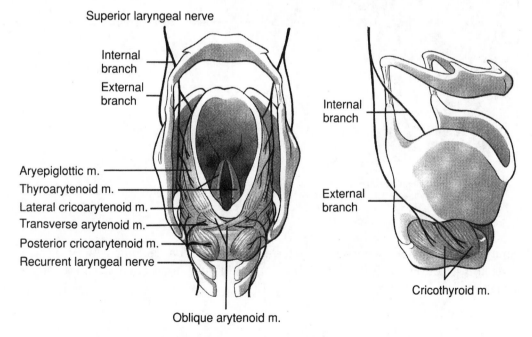

Superior laryngeal nerve

Internal branch
External branch

Internal branch

External branch

Aryepiglottic m.
Thyroarytenoid m.
Lateral cricoarytenoid m.
Transverse arytenoid m.
Posterior cricoarytenoid m.
Recurrent laryngeal nerve

Cricothyroid m.

Oblique arytenoid m.

Figure 3–3. Innervation of the larynx including central nervous system. Note the course and branches of CN X. Although not shown, the L RLN descends deep into the chest, looping under the aorta before ascending to the laryngeal region. From *The Pediatric Airway* by C. M. Myer III, R.T. Cotton, and S. R. Schott, 1995. Adapted with permission from Lippincott, Williams & Wilkins.

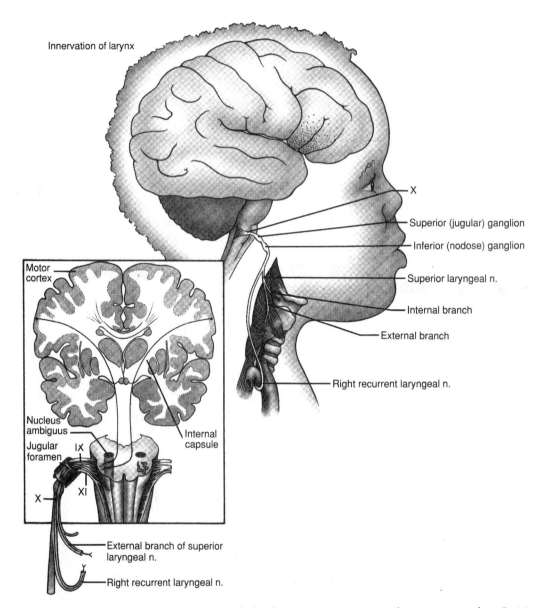

Innervation of larynx

X

Superior (jugular) ganglion

Inferior (nodose) ganglion

Superior laryngeal n.

Internal branch

External branch

Right recurrent laryngeal n.

Motor cortex

Nucleus ambiguus

Internal capsule

Jugular foramen

IX

X

XI

External branch of superior laryngeal n.

Right recurrent laryngeal n.

Figure 3–4. Peripheral innervation of the larynx. From *The Pediatric Airway* by C. M. Myer III, R.T. Cotton, and S. R. Schott, 1995. Reprinted with permission from Lippincott, Williams & Wilkins.

The main trunks of both vagus nerves descend deep into the gut and bring with them sympathetic and parasympathetic fibers of the autonomic nervous system (ANS) for innervation of viscera. These digestive structures include the following: alimentary canal, stomach, small and large intestines, and part of the colon; liver, pancreas, and heart via their sympathetic and parasympathetic fibers, and part of the ANS (Kingsley, 2000).

Clinical Note on paralysis: The left RLN is more susceptible to injury because of its longer course. Diseases, masses, or iatrogenic trauma can injure the nerve resulting in paralysis of the left true vocal fold (TVF) paralysis. As such, a previously undiagnosed left TVF paralysis requires a medical evaluation that includes imaging from the skull base to and through the chest region. Premature infants who undergo a patent ductus arteriosus (PDA) ligation are at risk for iatrogenic injury, as are babies born with complex cardiac conditions requiring chest surgery.

Laryngeal and Pulmonary Reflexes

The respiratory and laryngeal reflexes are mono- or polysynaptic, automatic, physical, protective responses. Although healthy individuals have these reflexes, the degree of response can vary from person to person and be suppressed or heightened under certain health- or medication-related conditions, or over the lifespan. Laryngeal or airway protection reflexes and respiratory reflexes are mediated by various branches of CN X. Recall that glottic and supraglottic sensation are mediated by the internal branch of the superior laryngeal nerve, and infraglottic and tracheal sensation are mediated by branches off the RLN. Mechano- and chemoreceptors located in the larynx and trachea are the afferents responsible for signaling the presence of foreign material. All motor responses are by way of the RLN. Branches of the vagus nerve mediate both sensation and motor responses to and from the esophagus. Afferents in the esophagus respond to "acid and distention" (Rudolph, 1995, p. 329).

■ *Laryngeal adductor reflex.* This airway protection reflex is triggered by mechanical or chemical stimulation (e.g., touch) of the supraglottic larynx, the region served by the SLNib. In response to the stimulus, the TVFs will abruptly snap shut. This reflex can be tested by touching the aryepiglottic folds with the end of a scope or pressurized air pulse, as is done during fiberoptic endoscopic evaluation of swallowing with sensory testing (Aviv et al., 1999).

■ *Esophagoglottal reflex.* This reflex occurs when there is abrupt distention of the upper esophagus resulting in a rapid closure of the larynx. Also considered an airway protection reflex, this response will prevent regurgitated or refluxed material from entering the laryngeal and lower airway (Shaker & Hogan, 2000). This reflex is well documented in adults, and within the past decade has been identified in infants (Jadcherla, Gupta, Coley, Fernandez, & Shaker, 2007). Failure of the larynx to close during regurgitation or reflux can result in serious pulmonary health issues (Jadcherla, Hogan, & Shaker, 2010).

■ *Esophago–upper esophageal sphincter (UES) reflex:* This reflex is similar to the esophagoglottal reflex in that the UES tightens with distention of the esophagus in order to prevent a backflow of regurgitated or refluxed materials from leaving the esophagus.

■ *Laryngospasm.* This is an exaggerated laryngeal closure that is a reflexive response to stimulation of the glottic and supraglottic structures. This can occur when there is mechanical or chemical stimulation from foreign material (e.g., stomach acid, water) that enters the laryngeal airway.

■ *Spontaneous cough.* Spontaneous cough is a complex protective response. When a cough is stimulated, the motor response involves tight compression of the true and false vocal folds, which in turn permits an increase in subglottic pressure and the forceful expulsion of material (e.g., mucus) from the laryngeal and tracheal airways. It is important to note that the cough response is complex, in that it can be triggered by irritants in the laryngeal, tracheal, and bronchial airways, all served by branches of CN X.

■ *Choking.* This is a common term for when the larynx responds to the presence of foreign material. It is basically protective laryngeal reflexes trying to quickly rid the laryngeal airway of material and can result in a laryngospasm or asphyxiation if the airway is completely obstructed.

■ *Cessation of respiration/apnea during swallowing.* Cessation of respiration, also referred to as apneic pause, is a medullary brainstem–mediated reflex. During swallowing, there is rapid laryngeal closure to prevent swallowed materials from entering the lower airway. In coordination with this laryngeal closure, there is a brief pause in respiratory activity, so that no inhalation or exhalation occurs. This is a normal event and, while coordinated with the mechanical closure of the larynx, relies on an independent neural activity (Hiss, Strauss, Treole, & Boutilier, 2003). For example, respiratory-cessation pauses occur in individuals who have undergone a total laryngectomy (removal of the larynx) (Hiss et al., 2003). Durations of respiratory cessation during swallowing vary but in most infants and young children are typically less than one second. Some respiratory pauses are considered normal in premature and term infants, but frequent apnea suggests an immaturity or abnormality of this neural mechanism or a mechanism higher within the CNS. Problems arise when the duration of the respiratory pauses or apnea is abnormally long (1–20 seconds in premature babies). Apnea is triggered by threats to the airway. Such threats can include direct reflux of gastric acids and pepsins resulting in material contact with the laryn-

geal airway, or direct contact by some other foreign material such as water, a bolus, or object.

■ *Vagal.* The vagal or vasovagal response is an unexpected and abnormal slowing of the heart (bradycardia) resulting from altered neural inputs. Vagal output for viscera is by way of the dorsal motor nucleus of CN X in the medulla. There is a resulting change in cardiac blood volume and arterial diameter(s), resulting in lowered blood pressure. Sudden onsets can result in fainting. Generally speaking, two main types are described: A *central* vagal response is due to stimulation from the hypothalamus to the medullary cardiac centers in response to pain, extreme emotion, and/or stress; a *peripheral* vagal response can occur when there is a loss of central blood volume, which in turn triggers hypotension (van Lieshout, Wieling, & Karemaker, 1997; van Lieshout, Wieling, Karemaker, & Eckberg, 1991).

Pediatric Voice and Disorders of the CNS

Voice production disorders can occur when any of the CNS controls have been disturbed by various diseases, trauma, or anatomic anomalies, such as Chiari malformation (CM), cerebral palsy (CP), pediatric movement disorders, muscular dystrophy (MD), traumatic brain injury, cerebrovascular accident, or CNS neoplasms and their subsequent treatment. Voice or respiratory, phonatory, articulatory disturbances due to CNS damage or disease will generally correspond to the area of involvement and effects of medications used to improve or mitigate symptoms or chemo and radiation therapies. Following is an overview of primary CNS conditions that may produce voice or related functional disorders.

Chiari Malformation

CM is a congenital CNS condition where there is a defect in a neural tube and/or cranial vault (posterior fossa), resulting in crowding of the cerebellar and brainstem region. It is categorized by severity and associated complications. The categories are types I, II, III, and IV. Type I CM (CIM) is caused by herniation of the cerebellar tonsils that extends 3 to 5 mm below the level of the foramen magnum. It can be relatively silent, not producing any obvious symptoms. If silent, it is not uncommon for a CIM to be found incidentally during imaging for another complaint (Mueller, 2001). Alternatively, it can cause issues like headaches, numbness and tingling in the hands, and shoulder pain and imbalance if there is compression of the upper spinal and midlower cranial nerves and increased intracranial pressure. Possible speech and voice symptoms can include vocal fold paresis, paralysis, and oral motor deficits.

Diagnosed in utero or in infancy, types II–IV CM symptoms are immediately apparent and are due to some combination of anatomic defects such as greater displacement of the cerebellar tonsils and more extensive involvement of the brainstem, dilation of the central canal, increased intracranial pressure, presence of spina bifida, and direct compression or traction on CN rootlets affecting their function (Akbari et al., 2013). In the case of compression of CN X, there will be a corresponding unilateral or bilateral vocal fold paresis or paralysis. Other CNs in the lower brainstem can also be affected, resulting in corresponding symptoms with facial, pharyngeal, and even lingual function. Early neurosurgical decompression can relieve the compression on the CN rootlets, but that does not guarantee restoration of function. If there is bilateral TVF paralysis, a tracheotomy may be required to secure a patent airway. Oralpharyngeal and esophageal dysphagia and airway protection problems are likely comorbidities to any voice disturbance.

Cerebral Palsy

CP makes up the largest neurologic disorder of childhood. Attributed to CNS injury at or around the time of birth, the type and degree of CP become evident as the child fails to develop motor function in a typical fashion. The range of symptoms a child demonstrates reflects the extent and location of involved CNS structures and pathways. CP is considered a chronic or static neurologic disorder in that it does not progressively worsen, although functional changes occur over a lifetime (Tatla et al., 2013). Persistence of primitive reflexes, hyper- or hypotonia, sensory deficits, and cognitive-linguistic delays can also be part of the symptom complex. CP is primarily categorized by clinical description of the type of persistent motor disturbances displayed: spastic, ataxic, athetotic, or mixed. Spastic CP is associated with involvement of the motor cortex and pyramidal pathways, resulting in high tone and limited or impaired acquisition of skilled motor movements. Athetotic CP is associated with extrapyramidal pathway involvement and as such results in poorly coordinated skilled motor movements and the presence of extra movements. Ataxic CP is associated with cerebellar dysfunction, with symptoms that reflect difficulty with coordinated movements and balance. Mixed-type CP involves some combination of the aforementioned types.

Disturbances of voice production in children with CP are related to the larger issues they have associated with dysarthria, including posture and trunk stability, respiratory support, and the ability to accurately execute and coordinate rapidly timed, skilled movements associated with articulation and voicing. It is common for children with CP to demonstrate difficulties with intelligibility of connected speech associated with deficits of prosody, pitch, and loudness control and resonance. In some instances, voice is not treated separately but rather in conjunction with all the major motor- and speech-specific deficits, and the child often receives care from several educational, medical, and allied health specialties. Despite the chronic nature of CP, there is evidence that improvement in connected speech intelligibility can occur when children receive a program focused on improving voice supportive of connected speech (Puyuelo & Rondal, 2005).

Movement Disorders

Fortunately, movement disorders in childhood are relatively rare, but they can occur secondary to CNS injury (e.g., CP) due to trauma, infection, inflammation, medication, disease, metabolic disorders, degenerative disorders, structural anomalies, and even some psychogenic origins (Wolf & Singer, 2008). Associated with the location of damage and cellular type involvement, movement disorders are grouped by symptom and clinical presentation. They include spasticity, ataxia, dystonia, rigidity and bradykinesia, chorea and ballism, tics, myoclonus, tremor, hypotonia, and weakness. Tics are the most common type of movement disorder found in childhood (Sanger, Delgado, Gaebler-Spira, Hallett, & Mink, 2003). Onset and presentation of vocal tics can be random or seen with other movement disorders (chorea). They are often associated with diagnoses of obsessive compulsive disorder and attention deficit hyperactivity disorder (ADHD). As previously mentioned, the onset of vocal tics can also be related to use of Ritalin, a medication for symptoms of ADHD. Persistent tics and coughing can be a cause of irritation to the laryngeal apparatus and the vibrating edges of the vocal folds.

Movement disorders are generally described as falling into two broad categories: those having positive signs (extra movement) and those having negative signs (lack of movement). An example of a positive sign would be a resting tremor, myoclonus, dystonia, or tic, as mentioned above. A negative sign would be diminished skilled motor activity characterized by rigid and bradykinetic extremity movement (difficulty reaching, crawling, or walking) and any articulatory movements relying on the coordination of respiration, voicing, and speech. Vocal symptoms will include hypophonia in combination with hypokinetic dysarthria. This type of disturbance can be seen in pediatric onset of Parkinson disease, which is caused by a depletion of the dopaminergic neurons of the basal ganglia.

Dystonia is defined as "involuntary sustained or intermittent muscle contractions causing twisting and repetitive movements, abnormal postures or both" (Sanger et al., 2003, p. e92). The exact cause of dystonia is unclear, but it can occur secondary to hypoxic ischemic events that have diffuse cortical involvement or dopamine deficiency (i.e., reduced dopamine uptake) in the basal ganglia. As with other movement disorders, dystonia can be part of the CP symptom profile. A focal dystonia occurs (e.g., writer's cramp, blepharospasm) when groups of small muscles spasm and interfere with function. Spasmodic dysphonia is considered by many to be a focal dystonia (Blitzer, Brin, & Ramig, 2009). Rare in childhood, spasmodic dysphonia is characterized by a spasm of the vocal folds during phonation activity in either the adducted or abducted position, resulting in a tight, pressed vocal quality (adductor) or intermittent bursts of air during phonation (abductor) (Blitzer et al., 2009).

Hypotonia or low tone (decreased resistance to passive movement at rest; Sanger, 2003) is not formally classified as a movement disorder but is a disturbance of central-peripheral proprioception and or cranial/spinal motor neuron function resulting from some type of disease process or CNS involvement. Low tone is not the same as muscle weakness, but the two can co-occur. Postural stability of the trunk and head/neck rely on adequate core tone, so associated voice difficulty will likely result from inadequate or poorly coordinated respiratory support during phonation. Moreover, voice can be specifically impacted, particularly if laryngeal muscle weakness is part of the symptom complex.

Any CNS event, such as a cerebrovascular accident, traumatic brain injury, or neoplasm, can cause a disturbance in voice. In some situations it relates to medical management of patients, in that they may require tracheostomy and ventilation, or some needed medication that impacts voice. But any vocal disturbance or executive control over vocal motor control can be the result of cortical damage to the frontal lobes, pyramidal pathways, subcortical structures, cerebellum, and brainstem. When there has been frontal lobe damage involving the premotor cortex and/or motor strip, the motor planning and initiation of voicing can be so disrupted as to result in a laryngeal apraxia or some degree of paralysis. Subcortical, cerebellar, and brainstem damage yield different types of vocal symptoms, many of which have already been discussed. Disturbances of pitch shift and intensity control, as well as coordination with respiration and motor speech movements, are often associated with damage in these regions.

Voice and Autism Spectrum Disorder

Autism spectrum disorder (ASD) represents a range of chronic linguistic and social communicative impairments whose diagnosis is often made in early childhood. Clinical and published reports note that voice disturbances can sometimes accompany ASD. Associated voice characteristics typically relate to abnormal prosodic intonation patterns (F_0 range and variability; I_0 range and variability) and intensity modulation (e.g., loud talking) (Russo et al., 2008) in combination with linguistic differences. Importantly these vocal characteristics do not necessarily constitute a specific type of dysphonia or abnormality of the vocal (vibratory) mechanism. Rather, there has been speculation that vocal pitch shift and prosodic issues reflect larger concerns with differences in the auditory feedback and vocal motor controls of children diagnosed with ASD. Difficulty with auditory feedback may also subserve problems related to speech perception and decoding the intent and emotion in a linguistic unit that is in part relayed by the changes in F_0 over the course of an utterance (Russo et al., 2008). Although the exact neural correlates of ASD are unknown, prosodic alterations or abnormalities can be associated with both cortical and subcortical changes (Iverson & Wozniak, 2007).

Numerous investigators have attempted to study the acoustical features of the cry of children with known ASD (Esposito & Venuti, 2010; Russo et al., 2008; Ting Wang, Lee, Sigman, & Dapretto, 2007). In one such study, the investigators reviewed the recorded cries of young children (18 months) who were diagnosed with some degree of ASD with varying patterns of development (Esposito & Venuti). Despite some methodological issues, investigators concluded that the acoustical features of cry for children with ASD (or at high risk for ASD) had distinct features. High-pitched cries and increased pause durations were two of the main findings reported. Higher pitched cries are known to be perceived as more aversive by the listener, in this case parents and caretakers. This cry structure can cause uneasy and uncertain responses by the caretaker and thus alter even the earliest communication exchanges (Esposito & Venuti; Ting Wang et al., 2007).

Chapter Summary

In this chapter we reviewed how the central and peripheral neural controls associated with voice production are organized within the central and peripheral nervous systems. Vocalizations or voicing can be innate or the result of an exquisite series of learned skills. Some human laryngeal functions and vocal skills are similar to those exhibited in the mammalian and animal kingdoms. Others are unique to humankind. Meaningful, healthy skilled vocalizations and reflexive laryngeal mechanisms rely on intact systems. Although much of what we know about the neural pathways and corticobulbar controls comes from animal research, results from investigations using functional imaging in humans, lesion studies, and embryology significantly add to our knowledge. Disorders of the CNS or PNS can lead to difficulty with voice specifically or in combination with other motor speech disturbances. Several neurologic conditions with associated disturbances in voice were discussed.

References

Akbari, S. H., Limbrick, D. D., Jr., Kim, D. H., Narayan, P., Leonard, J. R., Smyth, M. D., & Park, T. S. (2013). Surgical management of symptomatic Chiari II malformation in infants and children. *Child's Nervous System* *29*(7), 1143–1154. doi 10.1007/s00381-013-2040-9

Aviv, J. E., Martin, J. H., Sacco, R. L., Thomson, J. E., Diamond, B., & Close, L.G. (1999). Laryngopharyngeal sensory discrimination testing and the laryngeal adductor reflex. *Annals of Otolology, Rhinology and Laryngology,* *108*(8), 725–730.

Blitzer, A., Brin, M. F., & Ramig, L. O. (2009). *Neurologic disorders of the larynx.* New York, NY: Thieme Medical Publishers.

Corballis, M. C. (2003). From hand to mouth: Gesture, speech and the evolution of right-handedness. *Behavioral and Brain Sciences, 26*(2), 199–260.

Esposito, G., & Venuti, P. (2010). Understanding early communication signals in autism: A study of the perception of infants' cry. *Journal of Intellectual Disability Research, 54*(3), 216–223.

Henriquez, V. M., Schulz, G. M., Bielamowicz, S., & Ludlow, C. L. (2007). Laryngeal reflex responses are not modulated during human voice and respiratory tasks. *Journal of Physiology, 585*(3), 779–789.

Hirschberg, J., Szende, T., Koltai, P. J., & Illényi, A. (2009). *Pediatric airway.* San Diego, CA: Plural Publishing.

Hiss, S. G, Strauss, M., Treole, K., & Boutilier, S. (2003). Swallowing apnea as a function of airway closure. *Dysphagia, 18*(4), 293–300.

Iverson, J. (2010). Developing language in a developing body: The relationship between motor development and language development. *Journal of Child Language. 37*(2), 229–261.

Iverson, J. M., & Wozniak, R. H. (2007). Variation in vocal-motor development in infant siblings of children with autism. *Journal of Autism and Developmental Disorders, 37*(1), 158–170.

Jadcherla, S. R., Gupta, A., Coley, B. D., Fernandez, S., & Shaker, R. (2007). Esophago-glottal reflex in human infants: A novel reflex elicited with concurrent manometry and ultrasonography. *American Journal of Gastroennterology, 102*(10), 2286–2293.

Jadcherla, S. R., Hogan, W. J., & Shaker, R. (2010). Physiology and pathophysiology of glottic reflexes and pulmonary aspiration: From neonates to adults. *Seminar in Respiratory Critical Care Medicine, 31*(5), 554–560. doi: 10.1055/s-0030-1265896

Jürgens, U. (2002). Neural pathways underlying vocal control. *Neuroscience and Biobehavioral Reviews, 26*(2), 235–258.

Jürgens, U. (2009). The neural control of vocalization in mammals: A review. *Journal of Voice, 23*(1), 1–10.

Kingsley, R. E. (2000). *Concise text of neuroscience.* Philadelphia, PA: Lippincott Williams & Wilkins.

Krueger, J. M. (1970). A spectrographic analysis of the differing cries of a normal two month old infant. *Nursing Research, 19*(5), 459–462.

Larson, C. (1988). Brain mechanisms involved in the control of vocalization. *Journal of Voice, 2*(4), 301–311.

Loucks, T. M., Poletto, C. J., Simonyan, K., Reynolds, C. L., & Ludlow, C. L. (2007). Human brain activation during phonation and exhalation: Common volitional control for two upper airway functions. *Neuroimage, 36*(1), 131–143.

Ludlow, C. L. (2004). Recent advances in laryngeal sensorimotor control for voice, speech and swallowing. *Current Opinions in Otolaryngology-Head and Neck Surgery, 12*(3), 160–165.

Ludlow, C. L. (2011). Central nervous system control of interactions between vocalization and respiration in mammals. *Head and Neck, 33*(Suppl.), S21–S25. doi: 10.1002/hed.

Luria, A. R. (1973). *The working brain.* New York, NY: Basic Books.

Miller, A. J. (1999). *The neuroscientific principles of swallowing and dysphagia.* San Diego, CA: Singular Publishing.

Mueller, J. (2001). Brainstem conundrum: The Chiari I malformation. *Journal of the American Academy of Nurse Practitioners, 13*(4), 154–159.

Myer, C. M., Cotton, R., & Schott, S. R. (1995). *The pediatric airway.* Philadelphia, PA: Lippincott Williams & Wilkins.

Oller, D. K. (2010). Vocal motoric foundations of spoken language—a commentary on Iverson's "Developing language in a developing body: The relationship between motor development and language development." *Journal of Child Language, 37*(2), 275–279.

Palaez, M., Virues-Ortega, J., & Gewirtz, J. L. (2011). Reinforcement of vocalizations through contingent vocal imitation. *Journal of Applied Behavior Analysis, 44*(1), 33–40.

Poletto, C. J., Verdun, L. P., Strominger, R., & Ludlow, C. L. (2004). Correspondence between laryngeal vocal fold movement and muscle activity during speech and nonspeech gestures. *Journal of Applied Physiology, 97*(3), 858–866.

Puyuelo, M., & Rondal, J. A. (2005). Speech rehabilitation in 10 Spanish-speaking children with severe cerebral palsy: A 4-year longitudinal study. *Pediatric Rehabilitation, 8*(2), 113–116.

Rudolph, C. (1995). Gastroesophageal reflux and airway disorders. In C. Myer, R. Cotton, & S. Schott (Eds.), *The pediatric airway* (pp. 327–357). Philadelphia, PA: Lippincott Williams & Wilkins.

Russo, N., Larson, C., & Kraus, N. (2008). Audio-vocal system regulation in children with autism spectrum disorders. *Experimental Brain Research, 188*(1), 111–124.

Sanger, T. (2003). Pathophysiology of pediatric movement disorders. *Journal of Child Neurology, 18*(Suppl. 1), S9–S24.

Sanger, T. D., Delgado, M. R., Gaebler-Spira, D., Hallett, M., & Mink, J. W. (2003). Task force on childhood motor disorders classification and definition of disorders causing hypertonia in childhood. *Pediatrics, 111*(1), e89–e97.

Shaker, R., & Hogan, W. J. (2000). Reflex-mediated enhancement of airway protective. *American Journal of Medicine, 108*(Suppl. 4a), 8S–14S.

Simonyan, K., Saad, Z. S., Loucks, T. M., Poletto, C. J., & Ludlow, C. L. (2007). Functional neuroanatomy of human voluntary cough and sniff production. *Neuroimage, 37*(2), 401–409.

Smotherman, M., Kobayasi, K., Ma, J., Zhang, S., & Metzner, W. (2006). A mechanism for vocal–respiratory coupling in the mammalian parabrachial nucleus. *Journal of Neuroscience, 26*(18), 4860–4869.

Szaflarski, J. P., Rajagopal, A., Altaye, M., Byars, A. W., Jacola, L., Schmithorst, V. J., . . . Holland, S. K. (2012). Left-handedness and language lateralization in children. *Brain Research, 18*(1433), 85–97.

Tatla, S. K., Sauve, K., Virji-Babul, N., Holsti, L., Butler, C., & Van Der Loos, H. F. M. (2013). Evidence for outcomes of motivational rehabilitation interventions for children and adolescents with cerebral palsy. *American Academy for Cerebral Palsy and Developmental Medicine Systematic Review, 55*(7), 593–601.

Ting Wang, A., Lee, S. S., Sigman, M., & Dapretto, M. (2007). Reading affect in the face and voice: Neural correlates of interpreting communicative intent in children and adoles-cents with autism spectrum disorders. *Archives of General Psychiatry, 64*(6), 698–708.

van Lieshout, J. J., Wieling, W., & Karemaker, J. M. (1997). Neural circulatory control in vasovagal syncope. *Pacing Clinical Electrophysiology, 20*(3 Pt. 2), 753–763.

van Lieshout, J. J., Wieling, W., Karemaker, J. M., & Eckberg, D. L. (1991). The vasovagal response. *Clinical Science, 81*(5), 575–586.

Wolf, D., & Singer, H. (2008). Pediatric movement disorders: An update. *Current Opinion in Neurology, 21*(4), 491–496. doi:10.1097/WCO.0b013e328307bf1c

CHAPTER 4

Etiology and Management of Pediatric Voice Disorders

Contributed by Alessandro de Alarcon

Introduction

Pediatric voice disorders comprise a broad spectrum of problems commonly encountered in the clinical otolaryngology setting. The reported incidence of these disorders varies significantly, depending on data collection methods and the various pediatric populations sampled across different geographic regions (Wynne & Cohen, 2012); estimates range from 2% to as high as 23% (Boyle, 2000; Deal, McLain, & Suddarth, 1976; Silverman & Zimmer, 1975). Chronic voice disorders are known to impact social, psychological, and educational development as well as overall quality of life. In view of these potential problems, it is imperative for speech-language pathologists to have a sound working knowledge of the etiologies that contribute to the development of voice disorders and how they are best managed. This chapter presents an overview of this content.

Pediatric Voice Disorders: Risk Factors and Symptoms

Table 4–1 enumerates medical, physical, and behavioral risk factors that can precede, ac-

company, or follow voice change, as well as specific voice-change characteristics. Any child with voice loss or a change in voice quality should be referred to a pediatric otolaryngologist and a voice care team.

Specific symptoms of a childhood voice disorder can include any notable voice change that is distinctly different from age-/gender-matched peers, such as those displayed in Table 4–2.

Common Vocal Fold Pathologies

Vocal Fold Nodules, Cysts, and Polyps

Vocal fold nodules are the most commonly encountered cause of pediatric dysphonia (5%–40%) (Akif Kilic, Okur, Yildirim, & Guzelsoy, 2004). They are subepithelial lesions that may be intimately involved with overlying mucosa and are composed of thickened tissue similar in appearance to a callus. They generally do not involve the underlying superficial lamina propria. Because these lesions generally occur in children with heavy voice use or vocal misuse, it is thought that they arise as a result of repeated trauma. Presenting symptoms may include a chronic harsh

Table 4–1. Risk Factors Associated with Childhood Voice Disorders

Medical-Physical Risk Factors	*Behavioral Risk Factors*
A history or presence of:	A history or presence of:
■ Prolonged intubation	■ Vocal performance (e.g., plays, choir)
■ Tracheostomy tube	■ Athletic activity (e.g., cheering)
■ Laryngeal cleft	■ Vocal overactivity
■ Congenital aerodigestive disorder	■ Shouting
■ Arnold Chiari malformation	■ Yelling
■ CNS disorder	■ Screaming
■ Gastroesophageal reflux disease Eosinophilic esophagitis	■ Constant throat clearing
■ Lower airway disease (asthma, bronchopulmonary dysplasia, cystic fibrosis)	■ Harsh vocalization during play
	■ Poor diet choices/hydration
	■ Excess caffeine
■ Allergies	■ High fat
■ Connective tissue disease	■ High acid
■ Frequent upper airway infections	■ Low clear fluid intake
■ Craniofacial anomalies	■ Smoking or smoke exposure
■ Multiple medications	■ Alcohol consumption
■ Swallowing problems	■ Drug use
■ Upper/lower airway obstruction	■ Psychological disorder
■ Psychological disorder	

Table 4–2. Symptoms of a Childhood Voice Disorder

■ Hoarseness	■ Notable, persistent voice change after athletic performance and/or social activity
■ Breathiness	
■ Harsh, raspy sound	■ Chronic cough/throat clearing
■ Pitch that is too high	■ Change in swallowing
■ Pitch that is too low	■ Difficulty breathing
■ Voice that is too loud	■ Pain when voicing
■ Voice that is too soft	■ Psychological difficulty or trauma
■ Weak or high-pitched cry	■ Teachers or peers reporting difficulty understanding the child
■ Variable voice quality	
■ Voice loss	■ Change in social interaction and/or classroom participation

or breathy voice over a long duration. There also may be periods of aphonia, due to swelling of the vocal folds during extreme overuse. Nevertheless, there is usually no pain associated with voicing. Endoscopic examination often reveals fairly symmetric bilateral lesions in the midmembranous vocal fold. During vocal fold closure, a typical hourglass closure configuration is often seen. The size and location of vocal fold nodules variably affect mucosal wave, vocal fold vibration, and pitch (Plate 1). The perceptual assessment of voice quality varies from mild to severe dysphonia (Nuss, Ward, Huang, Volk, & Woodnorth, 2010 Tezcaner, Ozgursoy, Sati, & Dursun, 2010).

Vocal fold cysts are less common than nodules. They can be mucous or epithelial, and their location can vary from fairly superficial to deep within the vocal fold. Vocal fold cysts may be congenital or may occur as a consequence of a traumatic event in which the epithelium involutes to create a cyst within the vocal fold. Children with congenital vocal fold cysts usually have a history of dysphonia since birth, whereas those with acquired cysts may develop symptoms once the cyst is large enough to create a dysphonic voice. Presenting symptoms are generally similar to those of vocal fold nodules. Endoscopic examination often demonstrates a large unilateral lesion and a smaller contralateral reactive lesion (Plate 2). As with vocal fold nodules, the size and location of vocal fold cysts are frequently related to the effect on voice.

Like cysts, vocal fold polyps are less common than vocal fold nodules. These lesions are often exophytic, more pedunculated, and may have an obvious vascular supply and a related vascular ectasia. They are usually associated with an acute, memorable phonotraumatic event or chronic voice misuse. Some patients may, however, present with complaints similar to those in patients with vocal fold nodules or cysts. Endoscopic examination often reveals a lesion that is polypoid in appearance on the medial aspect of the vocal fold (Plate 3). There is typically an associated vascular ectasia or significantly increased vascularity of the affected vocal fold. If a recent acute hemorrhage has occurred, there will be evidence of extravasated blood in the affected vocal fold.

Management

The management of children with vocal fold nodules, cysts, and polyps frequently begins with a course of voice therapy with a speech-language pathologist with special expertise in pediatric dysphonia (Hersan & Behlau, 2000; McMurray, 2003; Tezcaner et al., 2009). Children who are 4 years of age or older and developmentally normal can generally participate in voice therapy. For younger children or those who are developmentally delayed or unable to participate in voice therapy, reassurance, vocal hygiene counseling, and routine office follow-up visits may be more advantageous. Voice therapy usually consists of 10 to 12 sessions over several months. Upon completion of this protocol, we recommend reevaluating the child to assess actual voice changes as well as both the parent's and child's perceptions of voice changes.

The speech-language pathologist plays a key role in relaying information pertaining to compliance with voice therapy to the surgeon. This information serves as an indicator of the feasibility of a successful surgical intervention, if needed. Operative management may be considered for children who show minimal or no improvement in voice quality after a course of voice therapy. Children who are compliant with voice therapy and able to integrate behavioral change into everyday life, but who have not made progress, are generally appropriate candidates for surgery. Children who are unable to incorporate change or who are noncompliant are also unlikely to comply with the demands of postoperative voice therapy and a mandatory period of voice rest. As such, these children are more likely to have recurrence of a lesion or a poor surgical outcome. The operative approach may consist of an endoscopy to confirm the diagnosis or to determine the possible esophageal contribution to the disorder.

Studies comparing nonoperative and operative management are limited (Mortensen, Schaberg, & Woo, 2010), and surgical removal of pediatric vocal fold lesions remains an area requiring further investigation. Patients with vocal fold cysts and polyps are more likely to undergo surgical removal, as both cysts and polyps are less likely to resolve nonoperatively. The decision to have a child undergo elective surgery should be made jointly by the surgeon, the child, and the caregivers. Children who are compliant with medical therapy, who have a significantly compromised voice-related quality of life, and who have no significant comorbidities that may affect surgical outcome are appropriate surgical candidates. Children who are compromised in their ability to communicate, have difficulty performing (i.e., singing or speaking in the classroom), and have experienced social repercussions are more likely to pursue surgical intervention. For children who meet these criteria but are uncooperative or noncompliant, a decision to delay surgery may be prudent.

Surgery should be performed by a pediatric otolaryngologist with special training in microflap techniques, and high-magnification microscopy and microlaryngeal instrumentation should be used to excise the lesion. Excision should be performed with the aim of maximally preserving the superficial lamina propria and normal vocal fold architecture. The pediatric laryngologist at our institution advocates using subepithelial infusion techniques together with microflap surgery to preserve the superficial lamina propria

(Hochman & Zeitels, 2000). After performing initial endoscopy, the child is placed in suspension laryngoscopy, and an operating microscope is used to visualize the vocal folds under high magnification.

Typically, the surgical incision is placed just lateral to the lesion and in parallel with the vocal fold. Sterile saline or a saline-epinephrine solution (1:100,000) is injected into the superficial lamina propria. This injection provides the surgeon with information regarding the location of the lesion within the vocal fold and expands the superficial lamina propria; this allows for a larger surgical space and decreases surgical injury and error. If lesions are bilateral, the worse side is approached initially. If there is concern about surgical healing or an aspect of the dissection that may lead to a worse voice outcome, the surgeon may elect to operate on one side only.

After injection is performed and the incision is made, dissection is carried out using microinstruments to expose the lesion. Vocal fold nodules are frequently subepithelial or intimately involved with the overlying mucosa; therefore, in some cases, the involved overlying mucosa is excised. Vocal fold cysts can occur in various locations and may be filled with mucosa-like material or epithelial debris. The key to achieving the best long-term results is to avoid the possibility of cyst rupture during removal by removing the sac of the cyst as well as the cyst contents. Vocal fold polyps are frequently associated with a hemorrhagic component and a prominent vascular ectasia. These ectasias should be treated simultaneously. The preference of the pediatric laryngologist at our institution is to ablate the ectasias using the potassium titanyl phosphate (KTP) fiber-based laser at its lowest setting. The polyp can be removed either by making a microflap and removing redundant tissue or by transecting the polyp off the surface of the vocal fold. After completion of removal, an additional subepithelial infusion is often performed. This informs the surgeon about the preservation of the superficial lamina.

The timing of surgery in children is often dictated by the need for postoperative voice rest and how this may affect the child's school schedule. In view of these considerations, surgery is often performed during the summer or during holiday breaks. Relative contraindications to surgery include uncontrolled medical comorbidities, such as gastroesophageal reflux or eosinophilic esophagitis, poor compliance with voice therapy, significant vocal abuse, and poorly controlled asthma or allergies.

Vocal Process Granulomas

Vocal process granulomas are uncommon in children and tend to be associated with intubation injury. Granulomas are areas where granulation tissue and inflammation create a growth on the medial aspect of the vocal process (Figure 4–1). This is the area that the tracheal tube in an intubated patient will rub against, creating initial injury and an inflammatory process. In patients who have not been intubated, there may be a history of a traumatic event that has led to injury of the vocal process and secondary development of the granuloma due to repeated trauma (e.g., phonotrauma, coughing, throat clearing). Symp-

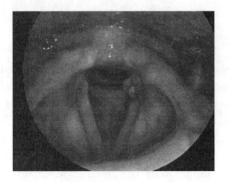

Figure 4–1. Left vocal process granuloma.

toms may include chronic coughing, chronic throat clearing, and throat pain. Perceptually, many patients exhibit borderline-normal voice quality. Large granulomas can cause significant voice problems by preventing vocal fold closure, which results in a breathy dysphonia. Endoscopic examination reveals a vocal process lesion that is often unilateral; hyperfunction of the lateral cricoarytenoid muscle is also frequently seen.

Management

The management of vocal process granulomas frequently involves voice therapy to address vocal hyperfunction. In addition to voice therapy, a proton-pump inhibitor and administration of oral steroids are often prescribed. These therapies decrease arytenoid inflammation at the granuloma site, frequently resolving the problem without the need for surgery.

For patients who fail this approach or who have airway obstruction secondary to the granuloma, surgical removal is indicated. This is accomplished by placing the patient in suspension microlaryngoscopy and using cold microlaryngeal instruments or the microdebrider to remove the granuloma. For children who have undergone multiple surgeries or for cases in which there is concern for potential recurrence, an injection of botulinum toxin into the vocal fold should be considered (Damrose & Damrose, 2008; Orloff & Goldman, 1999). This allows the surgical wound to heal without repeated trauma from vocal fold closure by paralyzing the vocal fold.

Vocal Fold Paralysis

Unilateral Vocal Fold Paralysis

The true incidence of both unilateral and bilateral vocal fold paralysis is unknown;

however, unilateral paralysis is more common than bilateral paralysis; and because of the longer course of the left recurrent laryngeal nerve, left-sided paralysis is more common than right-sided paralysis (Plate 4; McMurray, 2000, 2003). Iatrogenic injury leading to a vocal fold paralysis is much more common in children than in adults. The medical history may reveal severe upper respiratory infection, patent ductus arteriosus ligation, congenital heart surgery, anterior approach cervical spine surgery, thyroid surgery, mediastinal surgery, tracheoesophageal repair, or airway surgery (i.e., tracheal resection or cricotracheal resection). Children with decreased pulmonary function or those who have undergone recent cardiac surgery are unlikely to compensate for aspiration caused by the paralysis. Children with malignancies along the course of the recurrent laryngeal nerve may present with unilateral vocal fold paralysis caused either by pressure on the nerve or direct nerve involvement. Additionally, several case reports suggest an association between vocal fold paralysis and the chemotherapeutic agent vincristine (Burns & Shotton, 1998; Kuruvilla, Perry, Wilson, & El-Hakim, 2009).

Associated symptoms are typically a weak or breathy cry or a breathy voice quality. Some patients have diplophonia (two voice pitch sounds). To improve glottic closure, some patients compensate by using higher-pitched speech. Other patients have frequent bouts of pneumonia or coughing and choking with the ingestion of liquids, which is consistent with aspiration. Dyspnea during speech may be a common complaint; however, this is generally breathlessness and air hunger related to the loss of airway resistance during phonation.

Endoscopy and stroboscopy will reveal the paralytic vocal fold. The vocal fold can be in various positions, which will affect the severity of the vocal disorder. If the vocal fold is in the median position and there is good voice, there is typically a normal mucosal wave, good closure, and long phonatory segments during stroboscopy. If the vocal fold is in the paramedian or lateral position, stroboscopy may reveal chaotic vibration, poor glottal closure, and short-duration phonatory segments (Plate 4). The arytenoid may cause some hooding if it is tilted forward. It may also be rotated and lateralized, causing a large posterior gap. The position of the fold during phonation and the arytenoid position should be noted during the endoscopic examination, as both can play a role in treatment decisions.

Laryngeal electromyography (LEMG) evaluates electrophysiologic activity in the larynx and may offer useful information regarding the likelihood of the return of purposeful vocal fold function. Additionally, it may help in determining the location of the nerve injury. The reported prognostic value of LEMG in adults is variable; however, the utilization of discrete LEMG criteria improves the accuracy of prognosis for the recovery of vocal fold motion (Stratham, Rosen, Smith, & Munin, 2010). In children, difficulty in electrode placement because of tolerance levels and smaller muscle size is a limitation. In view of this, the role of LEMG in the evaluation of pediatric vocal fold paralysis has not yet been established and is currently being studied (Scott, Chong, Randolph, & Hartnick, 2008).

Management

Treatment of glottal insufficiency is generally determined by patients' symptoms, including the adequacy of their cough, the presence of aspiration, and the degree of phonatory dysfunction. Management strategies include observation, the use of temporizing measures, and longer term therapeutic interventions. In patients with a minimal voice deficit and/ or no aspiration, observation alone may be used while awaiting possible recovery of vocal fold function. Temporizing measures may be used in patients with a more significant voice deficit and/or aspiration. These measures may include voice therapy or injection laryngoplasty. Several injectables with varying durations of effectiveness are available (Levine, Jacobs, Wetmore, & Handler, 1995; Patel, Kerschner, & Merati, 2003; Sipp, Kerschner, Braune, & Hartnick, 2007). These injectables include Radiesse® Voice Gel, Restylane®, and Cymetra® (shortest to longest acting, respectively). In most children, injection laryngoplasty is performed in the operating room; however, cooperative teenagers may be able to tolerate an in-office procedure. Longer term injectables include Radiesse Voice® and autologous fat (Cantarella, Mazzola, Domenichini, Arnone, & Maraschi, 2005). Some adult studies suggest that early injection (i.e., 3 to 6 months after initial injury resulting in paralysis), may lead to the decreased need for permanent surgical procedures to restore glottic insufficiency.

Injection Laryngoplasty

When undergoing general anesthesia, the child is placed in suspension microlaryngoscopy. The injectable is then placed into the paraglottic space of the paralyzed vocal fold lateral to the posterior third of the muscular membranous vocal fold (Cohen, Mehta, Maguire, & Simons, 2011; Sipp et al., 2007). The vocal fold is then medialized until it is in the midline or just beyond the midline. If needed, a second injection may be performed more anteriorly. A small suction or laryngeal probe may be used to smooth out the vocal fold and the injectate. In children younger than age 3 years, overnight observation is advisable to ensure that respiration is not compromised.

Data pertaining to long-term voice outcomes with the use of Radiesse Voice® in children are scant. This injectable should be used

with caution, as it can be improperly placed within the larynx. Furthermore, with all injectables, increased caution is warranted, as the pediatric vocal folds are small. Meticulous control and placement of an injectate is essential, as injection into Reinke's space will result in impaired vocal fold vibration and distortion of the free edge of the membranous vocal fold. Before proceeding with a permanent procedure to address glottic insufficiency, the child should be followed for 9 to 12 months to ensure that spontaneous recovery does not occur.

Permanent Surgical Options: Medialization Laryngoplasty

Permanent medialization laryngoplasty with Gor-Tex or Silastic is best reserved for children who have gone through puberty and who thus have a fully matured larynx (Link et al., 1999). Delaying this procedure until puberty decreases the risk of needing revision laryngoplasty. Because optimal voice outcomes are best achieved in patients who are awake, this procedure is typically performed in children who are older and more cooperative. Regardless of the material used for medialization, the margin of error is relatively small. The surgeon should be skilled in the technique that is most suitable for the patient.

The patient is placed under deep sedation at the beginning of the procedure and a local anesthetic is injected in the overlying tissues around the thyroid cartilage. An incision is made and dissection is carried down to the thyroid cartilage. A window is made through the thyroid cartilage to expose the paraglottic space (Isshiki, Morita, Okamura, & Hiramotoa, 2009; Isshiki, Tanabe, & Sawade, 2009; Netterville, Stone, Luken, Civantos, & Ossoff, 2009; Zeitels, Mauri, & Dailey, 2003). Gore-Tex or Silastic is then used to medialize the vocal fold. During this portion of the procedure, sedation is lightened and implant size is titrated to the voice produced by the patient and heard by the surgeon. If the arytenoid cartilage is also in a poor position, an arytenopexy or arytenoid adduction is performed prior to the medialization (Isshiki et al., 2009; Zeitels, 2000).

Permanent Surgical Options: Ansa Cervicalis to Recurrent Laryngeal Nerve Reinnervation with Injection Laryngoplasty

An approach that has recently gained wider interest for use in children is ansa cervicalis to recurrent laryngeal nerve reinnervation with simultaneous injection laryngoplasty. Although this procedure is controversial in adults, a recent randomized controlled trial suggests that it may be advantageous in younger patients (Paniello, Edgar, Kallogjere, & Piccirillo, 2011). The procedure leads to voice outcomes (captured via stroboscopic examination and perceptual evaluation) that are similar to those associated with medialization laryngoplasty. Although reinnervation does not result in return of vocal fold function, it may provide improved tone to the denervated vocal fold and lead to a better position of the paralytic vocal fold during phonation. Another potential advantage of this approach in children is that it may provide a durable, stable voice without an implant. Moreover, it is unlikely to interfere with laryngeal development. Although there are currently no large-scale studies using this approach in children, anecdotal evidence and case series suggest that it may be a viable long-term therapeutic option prior to puberty (Paniello et al., 2011; Smith, Roy, & Stoddard, 2008; Zur, 2012). Nevertheless, rigorous studies of voice and swallowing outcomes are needed to better determine its utility. Reinnervation does not preclude the use of medialization laryngoplasty at a later date if a satisfactory vocal outcome is not achieved.

The procedure requires an open neck approach with the child under general anesthesia and should thus be performed by a surgeon with competency in pediatric open neck surgery. A distal branch of the ansa cervicalis is found and transected at its insertion into the strap muscle. Next, the recurrent laryngeal nerve is identified and transected distally in the neck. A neurorrhaphy of these two nerves is then performed under high magnification with either an operating microscope or surgical loops. Good mobilization of the transected segments is essential to ensure a tension-free anastomosis.

Families generally describe significant improvement from simultaneous injection; this improvement lasts 2 to 3 months. It is followed by worsening of the voice as the benefits of injection diminish. Ultimate voice outcomes following reinnervation typically do not occur until 6 to 9 months after the procedure.

Bilateral Vocal Fold Paralysis

As with unilateral vocal fold paralysis, the true incidence of bilateral paralysis is unknown. It is, however, thought to account for 10% of congenital anomalies of the larynx (Holinger, Holinger, & Holinger, 1976). Although bilateral paralysis is sometimes associated with birth trauma, central nervous system abnormalities, and cardiovascular anomalies (Rutter, 2007a), most cases are idiopathic. Depending on the position of the true vocal folds, affected children can present with aspiration, stridor, airway obstruction, a strong loud cry, and a good voice. Endoscopy/stroboscopy will reveal the vocal fold paralysis with the vocal folds in the paramedian or median position. Also, inhalation collapse of the membranous vocal fold can frequently be visualized. It is often difficult to distinguish between bilateral paralysis, bilateral cricoarytenoid joint fixation, and posterior glottic stenosis on awake endoscopy; in this setting, operative endoscopy is therefore indicated.

Management

Management of bilateral paralysis always involves striking a balance in optimizing breathing, aspiration, and voice. Voice outcomes following any intervention have historically included a simple nonvalidated questionnaire or the surgeon's perceptions of the voice result. Important to note, parents' concerns regarding their child's airway obstruction often result in an underestimation of the actual impact of the voice disorder on their child.

Initial management is often based on stabilization of the airway. Children who have problems with airway obstruction early in life often have a tracheotomy placed to bypass the obstruction. Most surgeons advocate waiting at least 1 year from the initial onset of bilateral paralysis before performing a procedure to open the glottic airway, as spontaneous recovery may occur. If a child has a tracheotomy or if there are signs of airway obstruction and a decision is made to improve this, several options for improving the glottic airway should be considered. These include: (1) open vocal fold lateralization, (2) laser cordotomy with or without partial arytenoidectomy, (3) endoscopic vocal fold lateralization, (4) laryngotracheoplasty with posterior graft, and (5) phrenic rootlet to posterior cricoarytenoid muscle innervation.

The decision regarding the procedure to be used is at the discretion of both the surgeon and the family. To date, there is only one comparative study that examines the outcome of decannulation. The authors found that a laryngotracheoplasty with posterior graft had the highest single surgical success compared with other procedures; however, it also had the highest risk of postoperative aspiration (Hartnick, Brigger, Willging, Cotton, & Myer, 2003). The pediatric laryngologist at our institution typically discusses the options with families and allows them to help in making the decision regarding the surgical procedure.

Open Vocal Fold Lateralization

A complete laryngofissure splitting through the anterior commissure is performed. An incision is made over the vocal process. A portion of the vocal process and arytenoid is then excised. A permanent Prolene suture is used to lateralize the posterior remnant of the vocal fold, tethering it to the thyroid cartilage.

Laser Cordotomy

Using a suspension microlaryngoscopy technique, the vocal process and part of the arytenoid and vocal fold are removed with a laser; a CO_2 laser is preferable, although other lasers can be used (Plate 5). A stent is almost always placed to help hold the defect open while it heals (Lagier, Nicollas, Sanjuan, Benoit, & Triglia, 2009).

Endoscopic Vocal Fold Lateralization

The vocal process and the posterior portion of the muscular membranous vocal fold are lateralized by placing an endoscopic stitch through the suspension microlaryngoscopy approach. A small stab incision is placed on the outside skin, allowing access to deeper tissue and facilitating the tying down of the stitch, lateralizing the vocal fold (Lichtenberger, 2002; Mathur, Kumar, & Bothra, 2004).

Laryngotracheoplasty with Posterior Graft

A rib graft is harvested and carved in a keystone shape. The larynx can be approached either via an open or endoscopic approach. The posterior cricoid plate is divided. The interarytenoid muscle may also be divided at the time of surgery, per the surgeon's discretion. The posterior graft is then placed in the defect, widening the posterior glottis. The graft should extend at least to the level just above the vocal folds. The patient either is intubated or a stent is placed, per the surgeon's decision (Thakkar & Gerber, 2008).

Phrenic Rootlet to Posterior Cricoarytenoid Muscle Innervation

Reinnervation of the posterior cricoarytenoid muscles with a branch of the phrenic nerve has more recently been reported (Marie, 2010; Marina, Marie, & Birchall, 2011). A rootlet of the phrenic nerve is found and a cable graft, typically a segment of the greater auricular nerve, is used to form a conduit from the phrenic rootlet directly into the cricoarytenoid muscle. Although this procedure is the only procedure that may provide both a good voice and a good airway, efficacy studies in children have not yet been performed.

Laryngeal Webs

Congenital laryngeal webs result from a failure of airway recanalization during embryogenesis. In many children, webs extend into the subglottis (Plate 6 and Plate 7). Given that 40% of children with a congenital laryngeal web also have velocardiofacial syndrome, all children with congenital webs should be evaluated for this syndrome (Rutter, 2007b). Children with significant webs typically exhibit symptoms of airway obstruction early in life. They often have a weak cry and can be aphonic or mildly dysphonic. Some patients, however, have good voices and strong cries and are minimally symptomatic. The length

of the web can influence the vocal quality by altering voice pitch. Endoscopy reveals a web with variable thickness and vibratory qualities.

Management

Management of laryngeal webs is often focused on improvement of the airway. The thickness and the length of the web play a critical role in voice outcome following surgery. Treatment of thick webs often yields minimal voice improvement and, in some cases, may result in a worse voice. Postoperatively, the vibrating surface of the vocal fold is scarred and has poor vibratory characteristics. Treatment of thin webs often yields improvement in voice, as the postoperative vocal fold generally has better vibratory characteristics. Treatment of longer webs often has a positive impact on voice outcome, whereas treatment of shorter webs may result in only minimal improvement. Families should be counseled regarding these aspects of web management and should be advised as to specific management goals (e.g., airway improvement and/or voice improvement).

Webs are managed either endoscopically or with an open procedure (Goudy, Sauman, Manaligod, & Smith, 2010). Endoscopic management is usually reserved for thin webs and webs without a significant associated subglottic stenosis. Through the use of a suspension microlaryngoscopy setup, the web is divided with cold instruments. A thin Silastic keel is then placed and sutured across the anterior commissure. This prevents re-formation of the web. The keel is left in place for 2 to 3 weeks.

In an open procedure, the web is divided under endoscopic guidance, and a complete laryngofissure is performed. The edges of the web are then sutured down to prevent readhesion. A small anterior graft is placed in the subglottis to address the stenosis; however, it should not extend through the anterior commissure. A stent is placed to prevent re-formation of the web.

Recurrent Respiratory Papillomatosis

Recurrent respiratory papillomatosis (RRP) is an uncommon disorder that presents with two distinct time periods: in children younger than age 5 years and in adults 20 to 40 years of age. According to data from the RRP task force national registry for juvenile onset RRP, there is an estimated incidence of approximately 1.7 to 4.3 cases per 100,000 children and 1.8 cases per 100,000 adults (Derkay, 1995; Reeves et al., 2003). RRP is caused by human papilloma virus (the same virus that causes genital warts) and is associated with cervical cancer (Plate 8). The two most common subtypes, 6 and 11, have a low risk of conversion into carcinoma compared with subtypes 16 and 18, which are associated with a much higher risk of conversion. The lifetime risk of conversion to malignancy is 3% to 7 % (Hobbs & Birchall, 2004).

Although children with RRP frequently present with stridor, airway distress, or airway obstruction, a subset of children presents with hoarseness (Derkay & Wiatrak, 2008). These children often require less frequent surgical debridement. Children who present with dysphonia related to RRP often have a characteristic harsh, raspy voice with voice breaks and periods of aphonia. On endoscopy, papillomatosis is characterized by sessile or pedunculated frond-like growths, which can be seen anywhere within the confines of the larynx (see Plate 8, subglottis to supraglottis). The characteristically normal vocal fold structure is often obscured when there is vocal fold involvement.

Management

Management of RRP involves surgical removal of the papilloma. This can be done with various instruments, including the microdebrider, the CO_2 laser, KTP laser, pulse-dye laser, or cold microlaryngeal instruments. The preference of the pediatric laryngologist at our institution is to use the microdebrider for bulky disease and the KTP laser to remove remaining disease or less invasive disease.

The timing of the surgery is based on the child's symptoms. Patients typically fall into two categories: those with voice symptoms and those with airway symptoms. Most children present with the latter. Surgery is often planned at specific intervals to prevent serious airway obstruction. Adjuvant therapy is often used for children with severe disease, which includes those who undergo more than four procedures per year, present with significant airway obstruction, or have distal spread into the trachea and bronchi (Derkay, 1995). Although many different types of agents have been used for adjuvant therapy, the most commonly used is cidofovir, an antiviral agent that is injected locally (an off-label use) (Gallagher & Derkay, 2009). A serious drawback of cidofovir is its potential for dysplasia or carcinoma (Derkay, 2005). Avastin® (bevacizumab), a newer drug that is an antiangiogenic agent, has been shown to be efficacious in several studies (Best et al., 2012; Maturo & Hartnick, 2010; Zeitels et al., 2011) and is now being used with minimal to no side effects. Despite the promise of this new treatment, Avastin is not curative and there is a need for further research and development of other adjuvants to treat RRP.

To ensure optimization of voice outcomes, utmost care should be taken in using tissue-sparing techniques. When the papilloma is removed, the surgeon should be mindful of not exposing the vocal ligament and of maximally preserving the superficial lamina propria. To prevent webbing, the surgeon should be mindful of anterior commissure papilloma. Children with RRP show varying degrees of dysphonia following surgery. Despite the need for frequent surgical intervention, many of these children have surprisingly good voice outcomes (Chadha et al., 2010; Holler et al., 2009).

Laryngopharyngeal Reflux and Eosinophilic Esophagitis

The incidence of voice disorders stemming from esophageal disorders is unknown. The most common esophageal disorders associated with pediatric dysphonia are laryngopharyngeal reflux (LPR) and eosinophilic esophagitis (EE) (Block & Brodsky, 2007; Dauer, Ponikau, Smyrk, Murray, & Thompson, 2006). Children with these disorders generally present with chronic coughing, throat clearing, and globus sensation. These symptoms are often worse in the morning and may improve during the course of the day. The dysphonia is usually perceived as a rough, harsh-sounding voice. Voice quality fluctuates and typically worsens with voice use. Although endoscopic findings are often variable, they may include vocal fold edema, erythema, vocal fold nodules, interarytenoid pachydermia, pseudosulcus vocalis, and thickening of the vocal fold cover (Plate 9).

Management

Patients with a suspected diagnosis of LPR or EE are often initially managed with a proton pump inhibitor for 1 to 2 months. Parents should be advised that this medication must be taken on an empty stomach 30 minutes before a meal. Most importantly, it should be given at times that offer maximal convenience and consistency to both the parent and the child. Additionally, the clinician should discuss dietary and lifestyle changes with patients and their families.

When the dysphonia and related symptoms persist, the patient should be referred to a gastroenterologist for an esophagogastroduodenoscopy (EGD), impedance probe testing, and biopsies. These diagnostic tests will distinguish between LPR, EE, and other disorders. Optimally, otolaryngologists and gastroenterologists work collaboratively to manage these patients. For more detailed information regarding the management of patients with EE, refer to the cited references (Dellon, 2012; Fornari & Wagner, 2012; Goldani, Nunes, & Ferreira, 2012; Putnam, 2011).

Sulcus Vocalis and Vocal Fold Scar

Sulcus vocalis and vocal fold scar are extremely rare. Sulcus vocalis is a loss of the superficial lamina propria with subsequent attachment of the underlying vocal ligament. A vocal fold scar occurs when an injury to the vocal fold causes loss of the superficial lamina propria, and the epithelium becomes adherent to the vocal ligament.

Fundamentally, both lesions are caused by the loss of the layered structure of the vocal fold, specifically the lamina propria. Sulcus vocalis can be congenital or secondary to trauma (Sunter et al., 2011), whereas a vocal fold scar is always associated with an injury. Patients typically present with vocal fatigue, a harsh voice quality, and excessive use of accessory laryngeal muscles. Endoscopic findings demonstrate a nonvibratory segment of the vocal fold that may appear as a linear striation within the medial aspect of the vocal fold. Perceptually, children may have a mild to severe dysphonia. The effect of the lesion on voice quality is related to its location and size.

Management

The management of sulcus vocalis and vocal fold scar is one of the most challenging problems in laryngology. Although authors have suggested various surgical treatments, results are variable (Bouchayer & Cornut, 1988; Ford, Bless, & Prehn, 1992; Ford, Inagi, Khidr, Bless, & Gilchrist, 1996; Pontes & Behlau, 1993). There is presently no good alternative for surgically reconstructing this layer. In most cases, clinicians conduct an initial operative examination to confirm the sulcus or vocal fold scar and perform a saline infusion to attempt to break up any scar bands; however, this may offer only temporary benefit or no benefit. Determining optimal management strategies is an area of active research, and our group of surgeons is awaiting the documentation of further treatment modalities before offering intervention.

Chapter Summary

Pediatric dysphonia comprises a broad spectrum of disorders with varying etiologies. Optimally, patients are evaluated using validated assessment instruments, and conditions are managed by an interdisciplinary team. Current research is focused on attaining a better understanding of dysphonia and on developing definitive treatment algorithms. Select cases depicting the aforementioned etiologies can be found on the accompanying DVD.

References

Akif Kilic, M., Okur, E., Yildirim, I., & Guzelsoy, S. (2004). The prevalence of vocal fold nodules in school age children. *International Journal of Pediatric Otorhinolaryngology, 68,* 409–412.

Best, S. R., Friedman, A. D., Landau-Zemer, T., Barbu, A. M., Burns, J. A., Freeman, M. W., . . . Zeitels, S. M. (2012). Safety and dosing of bevacizumab (Avastin) for the treatment of recurrent respiratory papillomatosis. *Annals of Otology, Rhinology, and Laryngology, 121,* 587–593.

Block, B. B., & Brodsky, L. (2007). Hoarseness in children: The role of laryngopharyngeal reflux. *International Journal of Pediatric Otorhinolaryngology, 71,* 1361–1369.

Bouchayer, M., & Cornut, G. (1988). Microsurgery for benign lesions of the vocal folds. *Ear, Nose, and Throat Journal, 67,* 446–466.

Boyle, B. (2000). Voice disorders in school children. *Support for Learning, 15,* 15–17.

Burns, B. V., & Shotton, J. C. (1998). Vocal fold palsy following vinca alkaloid treatment. *Journal of Laryngology and Otology, 112,* 485–487.

Cantarella, G., Mazzola, R. F., Domenichini, E., Arnone, F., & Maraschi, B. (2005). Vocal fold augmentation by autologous fat injection with lipostructure procedure. *Otolaryngology-Head and Neck Surgery, 132,* 239–243.

Chadha, N. K., Allegro, J., Barton, M., Hawkes, M., Harlock, H., & Campisi, P. (2010). The quality of life and health utility burden of recurrent respiratory papillomatosis in children. *Otolaryngology-Head and Neck Surgery, 143,* 685–690.

Cohen, M. S., Mehta, D. K., Maguire, R. C., & Simons, J. P. (2011). Injection medialization laryngoplasty in children. *Archives of Otolaryngology-Head and Neck Surgery, 37,* 264–268.

Damrose, E. J., & Damrose, J. F. (2008). Botulinum toxin as adjunctive therapy in refractory laryngeal granuloma. *Journal of Laryngology and Otology, 122,* 824–828.

Dauer, E. H., Ponikau, J. U., Smyrk, T. C., Murray, J. A., & Thompson, D. M. (2006). Airway manifestations of pediatric eosinophilic esophagitis: A clinical and histopathologic report of an emerging association. *Annals of Otology, Rhinology, and Laryngology, 115,* 507–517.

Deal, R., McLain, B., & Suddarth, J. (1976). Identification, evaluation, therapy, and follow up for children with vocal fold nodules in a public school setting. *Journal of Speech and Hearing Disorders, 41*, 390–397.

Dellon, E. S. (2012). Perspectives in clinical gastroenterology and hepatology. *Clinical Gastroenterology and Hepatology, 10*, 1066–1078.

Derkay, C. S. (1995). Task force on recurrent respiratory papillomas: A preliminary report. *Archives of Otolaryngology-Head and Neck Surgery, 121*, 1386–1391.

Derkay, C. S. (2005). Cidofovir for recurrent respiratory papillomatosis (RRP): A re-assessment of risks [Editorial]. *International Journal of Pediatric Otorhinolaryngology, 69*, 1465–1467.

Derkay, C. S., & Wiatrak, B. (2008). Recurrent respiratory papillomatosis: A review. *Laryngoscope, 118*, 1236–1247.

Ford, C. N., Bless, D. M., & Prehn, R. B. (1992). Thyroplasty as primary and adjunctive treatment of glottic insufficiency. *Journal of Voice, 6*, 277–285.

Ford, C. N., Inagi, K., Khidr, A., Bless, D. M., & Gilchrist, K. W. (1996). Sulcus vocalis: A rational analytic approach to diagnosis and management. *Annals of Otology, Rhinology, and Laryngology, 105*, 189–200.

Fornari, F., & Wagner, R. (2012). Update on endoscopic diagnosis, management and surveillance strategies of esophageal diseases. *World Journal of Gastrointestinal Endoscopy, 4*, 117–122.

Gallagher, T. Q., & Derkay, C. S. (2009). Pharmacotherapy of recurrent respiratory papillomatosis: An expert opinion. *Expert Opinion on Pharmacotherapy, 10*, 645–655.

Goldani, H. A. S., Nunes, D. L. A., & Ferreira, C. T. (2012). Managing gastroesophageal reflux diease in children: The role of endoscopy. *World Journal of Gastointestinal Endoscopy, 4*, 339–346.

Goudy, S., Sauman, N., Manaligod, J., & Smith, R. J. H. (2010). Congenital laryngeal webs: Surgical course and outcomes. *Annals of Otology, Rhinology, and Laryngology, 119*, 704–706.

Hartnick, C. J., Brigger, M. T., Willging, J. P., Cotton, R. T., & Myer, C. M. (2003). Surgery for pediatric vocal cord paralysis. A retrospective review. *Annals of Otology, Rhinology, and Laryngology, 112*, 1–6.

Hersan, R., & Behlau, M. (2000). Behavioral management of pediatric dysphonia. *Otolaryngologic Clinics of North America, 33*, 1097–1110.

Hobbs, C. G., & Birchall, M. A. (2004). Human papillomavirus infection in the etiology of laryngeal carcinoma. *Current Opinion in Otolaryngology-Head and Neck Surgery, 12*, 88–92.

Hochman, I. I., & Zeitels, S. M. (2000). Phonomicrosurgical management of vocal fold polyps: the subepithelial microflap resection technique. *Journal of Voice, 14*, 112–118.

Holinger, L. D., Holinger, P. C., & Holinger, P. H. (1976). Etiology of bilateral abductor vocal cord paralysis: A review of 389 cases. *Annals of Otology, Rhinology, and Laryngology, 85*, 428–436.

Holler, T., Allegro, J., Chadha, N. K., Hawkes, M., Harrison, R. V. Forte, V., & Campisi, P. (2009). Voice outcomes following repeated surgical resection of laryngeal papillomata in children. *Otolaryngology-Head and Neck Surgery, 141*, 522–526.

Isshiki, N., Morita, H., Okamura, H., & Hiramotoa, M. (2009). Thyroplasty as a new phonosurgical technique. In R. C. Branski & L. Sulica (Eds.), *Classics in voice and laryngology* (pp. 534–540). San Diego, CA: Plural Publishing.

Isshiki, N., Tanabe, M., & Sawade, M. (2009). Arytenoid adduction for unilateral vocal cord paralysis. In R. C. Branski & L. Sulica (Eds.), *Classics in voice and laryngology* (pp. 541–544). San Diego, CA: Plural Publishing.

Kuruvilla, G., Perry, S., Wilson, B., & El-Hakim, H. (2009). The natural history of vincristine-induced laryngeal paralysis in children. *Archives of Otolaryngology-Head and Neck Surgery, 135*, 101–105.

Lagier, A., Nicollas, R., Sanjuan, M., Benoit, L., & Triglia, J. M. (2009). Laser cordotomy for the treatment of bilateral vocal cord paralysis in infants. *International Journal of Pediatric Otorhinolaryngology, 73*, 9–13.

Levine, B. A., Jacobs, I. N., Wetmore, R. F., & Handler, S. D. (1995). Vocal cord injection in children with unilateral vocal cord paralysis. *Archives of Otolaryngology-Head and Neck Surgery, 121*, 116–119.

Lichtenberger, G. (2002). Reversible lateralization of the paralyzed vocal cord without tracheostomy. *Annals of Otology, Rhinology, and Laryngology, 111*, 21–26.

Link, D. T., Rutter, M. J., Liu, J. H., Willging, J. P., Myer, C. M., & Cotton, R. T. (1999). Pediatric type I thyroplasty: An evolving procedure. *Annals of Otology, Rhinology, and Laryngology, 108*, 1105–1110.

Marie, J. P. (2010). Nerve reconstruction. In M. Remacle & H. E. Eckel (Eds.), *Surgery of larynx and trachea* (pp. 279–294). Heidelberg, Germany: Springer.

Marina, M. B., Marie, J. P., & Birchall, M. A. (2011). Laryngeal reinnervation for bilateral vocal fold paralysis. *Current Opinion in Otolaryngology-Head and Neck Surgery, 19*, 434–438.

Mathur, N. N., Kumar, S., & Bothra, R. (2004). Simple method of vocal cord lateralization in bilateral abductor cord paralysis in paediatric patients. *International Journal of Pediatric Otorhinolaryngology, 68*, 15–20.

Maturo, S. & Hartnick, C. J. (2010). Use of 532-nm pulsed potassium titanyl phosphate laser and adjuvant intralesional bevacizumab for aggressive respiratory papillomatosis in children: Initial experience. *Archives of Otolaryngology-Head and Neck Surgery, 136*, 561–565.

McMurray, J. S. (2000). Medical and surgical treatment of pediatric dysphonia. *Otolaryngologic Clinics of North America, 33*, 1111–1126.

McMurray, J. S. (2003). Disorders of phonation in children. *Pediatric Clinics of North America, 50*, 363–380.

Mortensen, M., Schaberg, M., & Woo, P. (2010). Diagnostic contributions of videolaryngostroboscopy in the pediatric population. *Archives of Otolaryngology-Head and Neck Surgery, 136*, 75–79.

Netterville, J. L., Stone, R. E., Luken, E. S., Civantos, F. J., & Ossoff, R. H. (2009). Silastic medialization and arytenoid adduction: The Vanderbilt experience. A review of 116 phonsurgical procedures. In R. C. Branski & L. Sulica (Eds.), *Classics in voice and laryngology* (pp. 545–556). San Diego, CA: Plural Publishing.

Nuss, R. C., Ward, J., Huang, L., Volk, M., & Woodnorth, G. H. (2010). Correlation of vocal fold nodule size in children and perceptual assessment of voice quality. *Annals of Otology, Rhinology, and Laryngology, 119*(10), 651–655.

Orloff, L. A., & Goldman, S. N. (1999). Vocal fold granuloma: Successful treatment with botulinum toxin. *Otolaryngology-Head and Neck Surgery, 121*, 410–413.

Paniello, R. C., Edgar, J. D., Kallogjere, D., & Piccirillo, J. F. (2011). Medialization versus reinnervation for unilateral vocal fold paralysis: A multicenter randomized clinical trial. *Laryngoscope, 121*, 2172–2179.

Patel, N. J., Kerschner, J. E., & Merati, A. L. (2003). The use of injectable collagen in the management of pediatric vocal unilateral fold paralysis. *International Journal of Pediatric Otorhinolaryngology, 67*, 1355–1360.

Pontes, P., & Behlau, M. (1993). Treatment of sulcus vocalis: Auditory perceptual and acoustic analysis of the slicing mucosa surgical technique. *Journal of Voice, 7*, 365–376.

Putnam, P. E. (2011). Management of children who have eosinophilic esophagitis [Invited commentary]. *Journal of Pediatric Gastroenterology and Nutrition, 53*, 129–130.

Reeves, W. C., Ruparelia, S. S., Swanson, K. I., Derkay, C. S., Marcus, A., & Unger, E. R. (2003). National registry for juvenile-onset respiratory papillomatosis. *Archives of Otolaryngology-Head and Neck Surgery, 129*, 976–982.

Rutter, M. J. (2007a). Congenital airway and respiratory tract anomalies. In D. S. Wheeler, H. R. Wong, & T. P. Shanley (Eds.), *Pediatric and critical care medicine. Basic science and clinical evidence* (pp. 506–509). New York, NY: Springer.

Rutter, M. J. (2007b). Laryngeal webs and subglottic hemangiomas. In J. M. Graham, G. K. Scadding, & P. D. Bull (Eds.), *Pediatric ENT* (pp. 211–222). New York:, NY Springer.

Scott, A. R., Chong, P. S., Randolph, G. W., & Hartnick, C. J. (2008). Intraoperative laryngeal electromyography in children with vocal fold immobility: A simplified technique. *International Journal of Pediatric Otorhinolaryngology, 72,* 31–40.

Silverman, F., & Zimmer, C. (1975). Incidence of chronic hoarseness among school-age children. *Journal of Speech and Hearing Disorders, 40,* 211–215.

Sipp, J. A., Kerschner, J. E., Braune, N., & Hartnick, C. J. (2007). Vocal fold medialization in children: Injection laryngoplasty, thyroplasty, or nerve reinnervation? *Archives of Otolaryngology-Head and Neck Surgery, 133,* 767–771.

Smith, M. E., Roy, N., & Stoddard, K. (2008). Ansa-RLN reinnervation for unilateral vocal fold paralysis in adolescents and young adults. *International Journal of Pediatric Otorhinolaryngology, 72,* 1311–1316.

Stratham, M. M., Rosen, C. A., Smith, L. J., & Munin, M. C. (2010). Electromyographic laryngeal synkinesis alters prognosis in vocal fold paralysis. *Laryngoscope, 120*(2), 285–290.

Sunter, A. V., Yigit, O., Huq, G. E., Alkan, Z., Kocak, I., & Buyuk, Y. (2011). Histopathological characteristics of sulcus vocalis. *Otolaryngology-Head and Neck Surgery, 145,* 264–269.

Tezcaner, C. Z., Ozgursoy, S. K., Sati, I., & Dursun, G. (2009). Changes after voice therapy in objective and subjective voice measurements of pediatric patients with vocal nodules. *European Archives of Oto-Rhino-Laryngology, 266,* 1923–1927.

Thakkar, K., & Gerber, M. E. (2008). Endoscopic posterior costal cartilage graft placement for acute management of pediatric bilateral vocal fold paralysis without tracheotomy. *International Journal of Pediatric Otorhinolaryngology, 72,* 1555–1558.

Wynne, D. M., & Cohen, W. (2012). The paediatric voice clinic: Our experience of 81 children referred over 28 months. *Clinical Otolaryngology, 37*(4), 318–320.

Zeitels, S. M. (2000). New procedures for paralytic dysphonia: Adduction arytenopexy, Goretex medialization laryngolasty, and cricothyroid subluxation. *Otolaryngologic Clinics of North America, 33,* 841–854.

Zeitels, S. M., Barbu, A. M., Landau-Zemer, T., Lopez-Guerra, G., Burns, J. A., Friedman, A. D., . . . Hillman, R. E. (2011). Local injection of bevacizumab (Avastin) and angiolytic KTP laser treatment of recurrent respiratory papillomatosis of the vocal folds: A prospective study. *Annals of Otology, Rhinology, and Laryngology, 120,* 627–634.

Zeitels, S. M., Mauri, M., & Dailey, S. H. (2003). Medialization laryngoplasty with Gore-Tex for voice resoraton secondary to glottal incompetence: Indications and observations. *Annals of Otology, Rhinology, and Laryngology, 112,* 180–184.

Zur, K. (2012). Recurrent laryngeal nerve reinnervation for unilateral vocal fold immobility in children. *Laryngoscope, 122*(Suppl. 4), S82–S83.

Color Plates

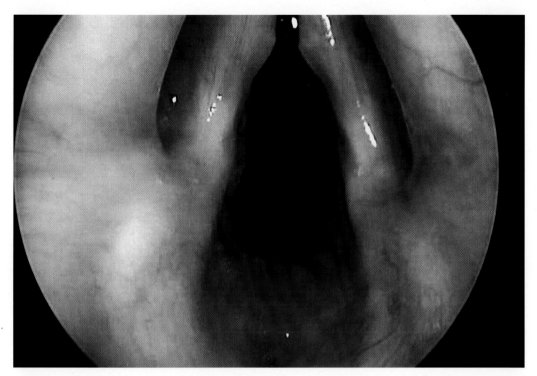

Plate 1. Nodules. Used with permission from the Center for Pediatric Voice Disorders, Cincinnati Children's Hospital Medical Center, Cincinnati, Ohio.

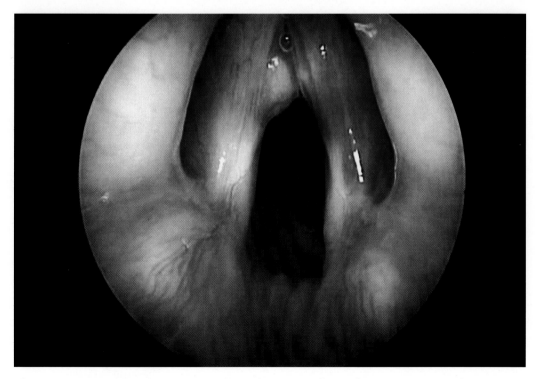

Plate 2. Cyst. Used with permission from the Center for Pediatric Voice Disorders, Cincinnati Children's Hospital Medical Center, Cincinnati, Ohio.

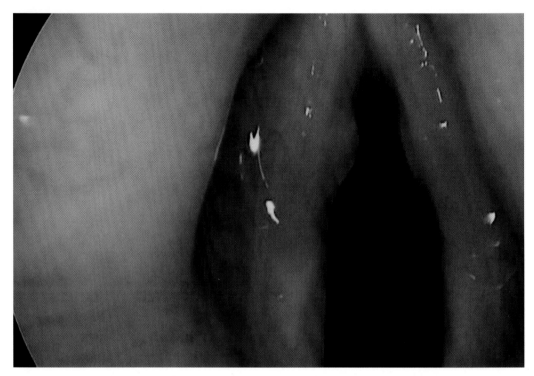

Plate 3. Polyp. Used with permission from the Center for Pediatric Voice Disorders, Cincinnati Children's Hospital Medical Center, Cincinnati, Ohio.

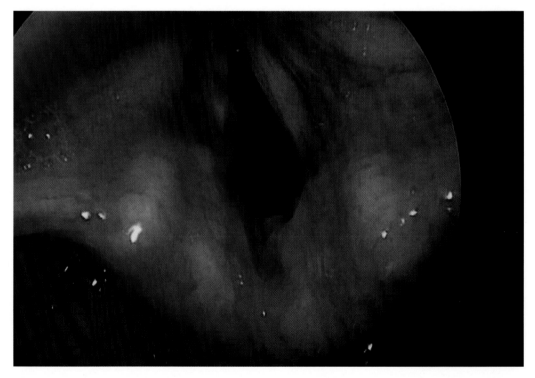

Plate 4. Unilateral vocal fold paralysis. Used with permission from the Center for Pediatric Voice Disorders, Cincinnati Children's Hospital Medical Center, Cincinnati, Ohio.

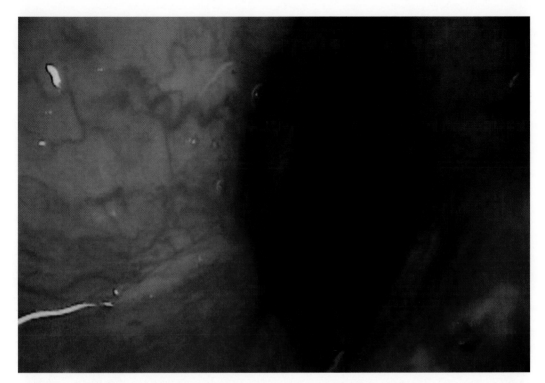

Plate 5. Cordotomy. Used with permission from the Center for Pediatric Voice Disorders, Cincinnati Children's Hospital Medical Center, Cincinnati, Ohio.

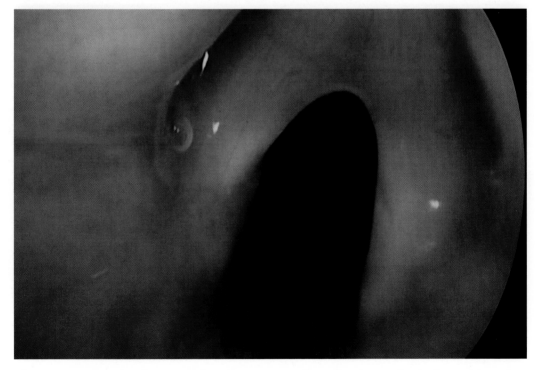

Plate 6. Laryngeal web #1. Used with permission from the Center for Pediatric Voice Disorders, Cincinnati Children's Hospital Medical Center, Cincinnati, Ohio.

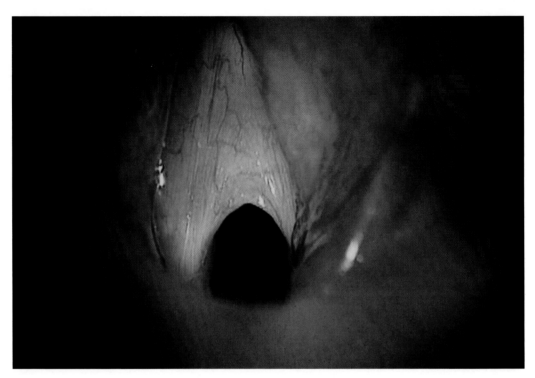

Plate 7. Laryngeal web #2. Used with permission from the Center for Pediatric Voice Disorders, Cincinnati Children's Hospital Medical Center, Cincinnati, Ohio.

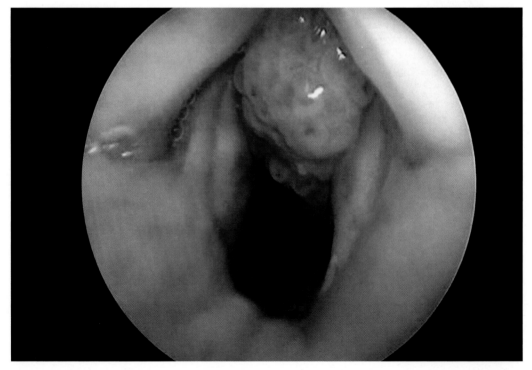

Plate 8. Recurrent respiratory papillomatosis. Used with permission from the Center for Pediatric Voice Disorders, Cincinnati Children's Hospital Medical Center, Cincinnati, Ohio.

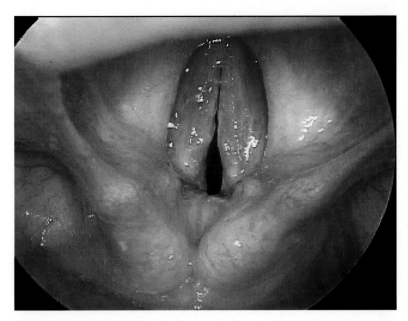

Plate 9. Physical (laryngeal) findings of supraesophageal reflux, vocal fold edema, and erythema. Used with permission from the Center for Pediatric Voice Disorders, Cincinnati Children's Hospital Medical Center, Cincinnati, Ohio.

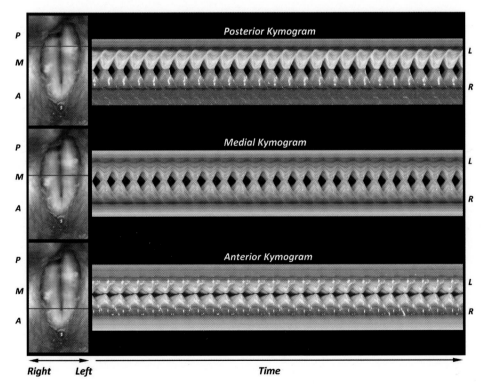

Plate 10. A point along successive vibration displayed via kymogram. Photo courtesy of Dimitar Deliyski, PhD. Communication Science Research Center, Cincinnati Children's Medical Center, Cincinnati, Ohio. Used with permission.

CHAPTER 5

A Collaborative Approach to Evaluating the Child with a Voice Disorder

Overview

This chapter discusses the available methods of pediatric voice assessment including initial interview, laryngeal imaging, perceptual analysis, acoustic analysis, aerodynamic measurement, and handicapping indices/quality of life instruments. These assessment areas will be covered with considerations for clinicians practicing in medical centers as well as from the standpoint of the solo and school-based practitioner.

The evaluation of a child with a voice disorder should not be treated as a "modified" version of an adult voice evaluation. Careful consideration must be paid to multiple factors such as the age of the child, maturity level, voice and speech capabilities, and the impact of dysphonia on daily life. Special planning is required and thoughtful consideration must be given to appropriate evaluation techniques and adaptive methods. The end result of the evaluation should be an identification of the vocal function components that are most impacted. Thorough documentation of laryngeal functioning prior to the initiation of therapy

is important for child/parent education, communication with referring physicians, and documentation for insurance reimbursement. An extremely important aspect of the evaluation is gaining an understanding of the impact of the voice disorder on the child's social and physical activities. The parent's/caregiver's perspective of that impact is essential to understand for treatment planning as well.

Evaluation Models and Approaches

Children may be identified as having a voice disorder by a variety of sources, including a caregiver, pediatrician, classroom teacher, or school-based speech-language pathologist (SLP). In many larger metropolitan areas, voice care teams who are prepared to complete voice evaluations with children are accessible to families. Often these voice care teams, consisting of, at a minimum, a pediatric otolaryngologist and SLP, become a referral center for a larger region with patients traveling several hours for the evaluation. In the scenario in which a child from a less urban area is traveling a distance for an evaluation, communication between the referral source and the voice care team is essential. Any details regarding the referral or previous evaluations of the child should be sent with the child/caregiver for the evaluation to assist in the diagnosis and treatment planning. The voice care team has an equal responsibility in communicating the results of the evaluation to the local treating clinician in the form of a report and perhaps video/still pictures of the larynx.

Many pediatric hospitals and medical centers have established collaborative evaluation teams involving pediatric otolaryngologists, SLPs, singing specialists, and often nurses to complete comprehensive examinations of speech and voice of children with dysphonia. Additionally, secondary players may greatly assist the management of the child, including an allergist, pulmonologist, neurologist, and psychologist.

An otolaryngologist is a physician who specializes in the treatment and surgical care of disorders involving the ears, nose, and throat (ENT). Otolaryngologists are often referred to as ENTs. In the evaluation of a child with a voice disorder, the otolaryngologist visualizes the larynx through endoscopic examination and determines appropriate medical treatments, such as medications, and in some cases performs surgery. Within the field of otolaryngology, there are additional subspecialists who treat specific disorders. For example, a *laryngologist* primarily treats disorders of the larynx.

The Solo and School-Based Practitioner with Otolaryngology Referral

There may be instances or clinical locations in which children are evaluated by an SLP prior to a medical examination by an otolaryngologist, such as in a private practice. In this case, the clinician should reserve any discussion of diagnosis of the voice disorder, as well as any treatment planning or initiation, until after the medical examination. Prior to the initiation of therapy, all children with a voice disorder must be evaluated by a physician (in most cases, preferably an otolaryngologist). The following statement is from the American Speech-Language Hearing Association:

> All patients/clients with voice disorders are examined by a physician, preferably in a discipline appropriate to the presenting complaint. The physician's examination may occur before or after the voice evaluation by the SLP. (ASHA, 2004)

The clinician can gather a case history and instrumental/perceptual information from the child/parent if completing the evaluation prior to the otolaryngology examination. Waiting for a medical evaluation is important. A clinician may strongly suspect that a child has vocal fold nodules based on his or her observation of phonotraumatic behaviors, report of laryngeal reflux-type symptoms, and perceptual quality of the voice. However, there is always the possibility that the child has a vocal fold cyst or, in a very rare case, a malignant mass on the vocal folds. Both of these lesions cannot be reduced in size or eliminated with voice therapy and require medical attention and potentially surgery.

In other situations, such as a school setting, the treating SLP has not participated in the evaluation, but rather is reading a diagnostic report from an otolaryngology practice or a pediatric voice care evaluation team. While the treating SLP may begin his or her role and evaluation of the child later in the evaluation timeline, knowledge of current procedures, instrumentation, and evaluation tools is helpful to the school-based clinician interpreting the report. It is the intent of the authors that this chapter provide both an understanding of how to obtain important measurements during a voice evaluation as well as an understanding of how to interpret the results.

Screenings

An SLP in a school setting may be asked to complete a screening of voice quality of an individual child or screen voice quality as a component of standard speech and language screenings (e.g., kindergarten entry screenings). Referral of a child with a voice disorder may be made to the school-based clinician by a parent or a classroom teacher. There are several published screening protocols for evaluating voice disorders in children, including the Quick Screen for Voice (Lee, Stemple, & Glaze, 2005) and the Boone Voice Program Screen (Boone, 1993). Both of these tools can easily be added to a standard speech and language screening performed in the school setting with kindergartners and/or new students.

The Quick Screen for Voice is a 5- to 10-minute protocol that evaluates the subsystems of voice production, including respiration, phonation, and resonance. The clinician listens to the child's voice by engaging him or her in conversation or a storytelling task. Additionally, there are several specific speech tasks that evaluate pitch range and maximum phonation time. In a report of the use of this screening tool in 3,000 elementary-aged children across 53 school districts in Ohio, 19% of kindergarten and first-grade students and 14% of fifth graders failed the screening (Lee, Stemple, Glaze, & Kelchner, 2004).

The Boone Voice Program Screening tool (Boone, 1993) is also a quick protocol that primarily assesses any deviance in pitch, loudness, quality, and resonance (oral and nasal). The s/z ratio is evaluated as well, which is described later in this chapter.

Both of these screening tools have a place on the form to indicate whether further

medical attention is required. These screening tools may be useful for documentation in a school setting.

The Medical Evaluation

As previously stated, every child who is referred for a dysphonia/voice disorder must undergo a medical evaluation, preferably with an otolaryngologist. The otolaryngologist seeks to identify the underlying medical precipitator of the disorder and whether any medical management is necessary (e.g., prescribing reflux medication, surgical removal of a lesion). The otolaryngologist will conduct a thorough ear, nose, and throat examination as well as perform palpation of lymph nodes and the thyroid. Basic visualization of the larynx can be completed with a laryngeal mirror, often referred to as mirror laryngoscopy. For this procedure, a small laryngeal mirror is placed at the back of the child's oral cavity and a light is shown on the mirror from a headset worn by the otolaryngologist. The advantages of this type of examination are that it can be completed quickly and without sedation/anesthesia. The disadvantages, however, are that the examination may be poorly tolerated by children due to a strong gag reflex and/or anxiety. Additionally, function of the vocal folds cannot be evaluated—only gross examination of the anatomic structures can be completed. More information about laryngeal visualizations/examination utilizing rigid and flexible endoscopes appears later in this chapter.

Oral Peripheral Examination

Another component of the medical examination is an oral peripheral examination, which assesses the structure and function of the face,

Table 5–1. Cranial Nerves

Cranial Nerve	Motor Function	Sensory Function
I		Smell
II		Vision
III	Movement of eyelid and eyeball	
IV	Movement of eyeball (laterally and downward)	
V	Mastication	Sensation of touch and pain to scalp, face, and mouth
VI	Movement of eyeball (turns eye laterally)	
VII	Facial expressions, secretion of saliva and tears	Sensation of taste in anterior two-thirds of tongue
VIII		Equilibrium and hearing
IX	Swallowing	Sensation of taste in posterior third of tongue, general sensation from pharynx and larynx, and sensation of carotid blood pressure
X	Phonation and swallowing	Sensation of pharyngeal cavity, thoracic cavity, and abdominal organs Two important branches: *Superior laryngeal nerve* Internal branch—sensations of the larynx External branch—innervation of cricothyroid muscle *Recurrent laryngeal nerve* Sensations below the larynx and innervation of all other intrinsic laryngeal muscles
XI	Movement of head and shoulder elevation	
XII	Tongue movement	

head, and oral structures. Specific structures examined are the lips, tongue, teeth, jaw, and hard and soft palates. The physical, anatomic structures are examined for any immediately observable deviations (e.g., facial droop, missing teeth). Motor and sensory functions of the primary structures are evaluated. These evaluations are important in children to identify any structural abnormalities that may contribute to or create a voice disorder. An evaluation of cranial nerves I through XII (Table 5–1) can also be included in this examination, particularly if a neurogenic cause is suspected. Evaluation of speaking rate and articulation may also reveal information about motor function of the head and neck structures.

Hearing Screening

Children who present with a voice disorder may benefit from an evaluation of their hearing ability. Due to the increase in newborn hearing screenings, many children with hearing loss are identified at a very young age. Approximately 50% of congenital hearing loss is caused by genetic factors (ASHA, 2008). Hearing loss can develop later in childhood, however, due to factors such as medication toxicity and noise exposure. Many voice care teams do not routinely screen for hearing loss; however, if elements of the medical/social history reveal that the child may be at risk or demonstrate signs/symptoms of hearing loss, a screening should be pursued.

Background and History

An initial interview with parent(s)/caregivers and the child will provide valuable details about the nature, history or timeline, and significance of the voice disorder. The SLP frequently has more time to explore potential contributing factors to the development or continuation of a voice disorder compared with other members of the evaluation team. Gaining a good understanding of the parents' goals and concerns at the beginning of the evaluation process will likely lead to an outcome and a plan of treatment that is more suitable to the family and the clinician. The following section describes areas that should be explored during a case history. In many clinical practices, the family may be asked to complete a case history form at home before the appointment or while they are waiting to see the voice team. Allowing for independent time to answer questions, particularly about the significance of the disorder to the child and family, may be enlightening for the clinician. A sample history form for use with a pediatric patient and her or his parent(s) is found in Appendix 5–1.

Significant Medical History

Due to laryngeal disorders that may occur as a result of prolonged intubation and ventilation, a complete medical history related to the child's birth, hospitalization, and discussion of previous significant illnesses will be important in the diagnosis. Caregivers should be queried regarding whether or not the child was premature and required assistance with breathing at birth. Based on etiologies of voice disorders found in children, other areas of interest include a history of any of the following: gastroesophageal reflux disease (GERD), eosinophilic esophagitis, respiratory disorders such as asthma and bronchopulmonary dysplasia, heart disorder or previous surgery, cancer, swallowing disorder, and any disorder affecting motor or cognition (head trauma, cerebral palsy, Down syndrome). The clinician should also probe for information about medications the child may be taking, such as antihistamines (which may have systemic dehydrating effects) or medications for attention deficit/hyperactivity disorder (ADHD), such as Ritalin, which have been found to produce vocal tics in children when prescribed in higher doses (Medline Plus, 2013). As GERD has such a strong potential to contribute to the development of vocal irritation and potentially lesions, additional probing questions should be asked of the child/parent if GERD is suspected, including questions about eating habits, increased hoarseness and/or phlegm in the morning, and/or bad breath.

Vocal Hygiene

Current care of the laryngeal mechanism is of interest to the evaluating clinicians. Due to potential harm to the tissue of the larynx, the following questions should be asked during the case history: (1) Is the child exposed to cigarette or other types of smoke or environmental toxins? (2) How much water or other liquids does the child consume each day? (3) How many caffeinated products does the child consume each day or week (e.g., soda, chocolate, coffee)? (4) Does the child exhibit any of the following behaviors in excess: screaming, crying, throat clearing, loud talking, or coughing?

plex histories related to intubation (prolonged or potentially emergent). Frequently, these children were premature and have other respiratory disorders related to problems with lung development. Therefore, it is appropriate for the evaluating clinician to ask questions about the following: (1) previous intubation and/or tracheotomy (including whether or not they were emergent and the number of procedures), and (2) symptoms of stridor, snoring, or shortness of breath (dyspnea).

Vocal Symptoms

It is important for the evaluating clinicians to understand the current symptoms the child is experiencing related to vocal function. Children in particular, due to shyness or fear of a medical examination, may not speak in a manner that is typical of everyday function during the formal evaluation. The caregiver can provide the clinicians with information regarding the following voice symptoms: loudness (too loud or soft), pitch (too high or low), hoarseness, breathiness, pain, effort, or fatigue associated with voicing. The timeline and pattern of vocal symptom onset is important as well.

> Clinical Note: A parent might report that the child has always been hoarse, which may be consistent with lesions such as a congenital cyst. A child/parent also might report a sudden onset after a heavy vocal performance schedule, which might be consistent with the development of a vocal fold polyp or vocal fold nodules.

Airway History

As previously stated, many children presenting with voice disorders have medically com-

Behavioral Questions

Information may be gained during the case history that will help the evaluating clinicians comprehend the child's ability to understand information about his or her voice disorder, as well as complete exercises and home practice related to voice therapy. These questions would include information about the following: (1) current academic progress/whether the child is performing at an age-appropriate grade level, (2) developmental delays, and (3) behavioral concerns (e.g., diagnosis of ADHD). Related to this area, the clinician may also want to ask older children/caregivers about activities that they are involved in, such as singing lessons, choirs, or sports that involve cheering.

Special Circumstances

Recommendations for working with a child who is singing and/or acting on a regular basis are discussed further in Chapter 6. In these cases, the clinician will want to understand as much as possible about previous training, current teaching methodologies, expectations for voice, and future plans. Evaluation and treatment of patients with functional disorders such as paradoxical vocal fold dysfunction also require specific questioning. More information and key history questions for this patient population appear in Chapter 7.

Assessing Impact: Handicapping and Quality of Life Indicators

There are currently several tools available to evaluate the impact of a voice disorder on quality of life in children. For children, these tools are typically completed by parent proxy, meaning that the parent completes the form. The completion of one of the available scales at the initial evaluation session will provide the clinician with valuable information about the impact of the voice disorder on actual voice use, as well as the social/emotional impact. Understanding the significance of the voice disorder will help the clinician understand the level of priority that voice improvement plays in the parent/child's life, as well as motivation for therapy. These tools should also be completed throughout a course of voice therapy to gain a better understanding of perceived progress and improved function. Table 5–2 provides the name of each tool and a reference in which a copy of the form can be found.

The first published parent-proxy quality of life tool directed toward pediatric voice disorders was the Pediatric Voice Outcome Survey (PVOS; Hartnick, 2002). This tool was first administered to children who had upper airway concerns and were currently tracheotomized or decannulated. The original tool had five questions, with one addressing swallowing concerns. In a subsequent study to further establish the validity of this survey, the number of questions was reduced to four (Hartnick, Volk, & Cunningham, 2003). The findings of the subsequent study found the tool to have acceptable internal consistency (Cronbach alpha = .70). Test-retest reliability was found to be in an acceptable range as well.

Table 5–2. Instruments for Measuring Perceived Impact of Voice Disorders in Children

Instrument Name	Reference
Pediatric Voice Handicap Index (pVHI)	Zur et al. (2007)
Pediatric Voice-Related Quality of Life (PVRQOL)	Boseley, Cunningham, Volk, & Hartnick (2006)
Pediatric Voice Outcomes Survey (PVOS)	Hartnick (2002)

A copy of the assessment tool is found in the text or the appendices of the articles above.

Another such tool is the Pediatric Voice Handicap Index (pVHI; Zur et al., 2007). This tool is an adaptation of the Voice Handicap Index (VHI) as a parent-proxy form. The tool is a 23-item survey with subscales focusing on functional, physical, and emotional aspects of voice disorders. The parent responds to statements such as, "My child's voice sounds dry, raspy, and/or hoarse" with a rating on a 4-point Likert scale. The tool also contains a 7-point Likert scale in which the parent rates the child's level of talkativeness. A normative data study including 45 parents of children with voice disorders revealed high internal consistency and test-retest reliability (Zur et al., 2007).

The Pediatric Voice-Related Quality of Life (PVRQOL) is another parent-proxy tool utilized for evaluating parent perception of the impact of a voice disorder (Boseley, Cunningham, Volk, & Hartnick, 2006). This tool has 10 statements to which parents respond about their child's voice using a 6-point Likert scale. Merati, Keppel, Braun, Blumin, and Kerschner (2008) examined the results of this tool in children with voice disorders compared with children with no known voice impairment. Comparison of scores revealed that children with voice disorders had significantly higher scores on this tool.

Perceptual Evaluation

Although the actual perceived quality of the voice is often the biggest "driver" in regard to referral, treatment decisions, and discharge from treatment, it is among the most difficult aspects of voice production to measure. Frequently, acoustic measures and underlying physiologic causes of a voice disorder do not correlate well with perceptual measurements (Shrivastav & Sapienza, 2003). Challenges in consistency of perceptions amongst individuals are highly dependent on factors such as the evaluator's age, gender, clinical experience, and cultural background. Several studies have examined the impact of level of experience with voice disorders on perceptual ratings and have found mixed results. Some studies have found that experience with voice disorders causes an individual to be more sensitive or "bothered" by the dysphonia and thus rate voices more severely (e.g., Damrose, Goldman, Groessl, & Orloff, 2004). Other studies have found that more experienced listeners rate less severely as they are more sensitized to dysphonia (e.g., Laczi, Sussman, Stathopoulos, & Huber, 2005). An aspect of this consistency not frequently discussed in the literature is calibration of an individual's perception. This consistency of rating is incredibly important for perceptual ratings of children who have a high likelihood of being evaluated and treated in two different clinical settings. Clinicians should take the time, particularly if they are frequently treating/evaluating patients who will be seen in other locations, to "check" their ratings against other professionals' (at their clinical location and in their region) to determine whether they are in line with common ranges of severity ratings.

Standardized protocols for the completion of perceptual evaluation are provided in the literature. Two of the most common protocols are the dysphonia scale for grade, *r*oughness, *b*reathiness, *a*sthenia, and *s*train (GRBAS; Hirano, 1981) and the Consensus Auditory Perceptual Evaluation of Voice (CAPE-V; Kempster, Gerratt, Verdolini Abbott, Barkmeier-Kraemer, & Hillman, 2009). Both of these scales require the clinician to evaluate the voice quality related to a set of perceptual characteristics after listening to the child's voice during the evaluation.

The GRBAS utilizes a 4-point Likert scale for the perceptual qualities of dysphonia it measures. Several studies in the literature have utilized this scale for children with voice disorders (e.g., Reynolds et al., 2012) and found it to reliably document improved voice quality in children with vocal nodules following a course of voice therapy (Tezcaner, Ozgursoy, Sati, & Dursun, 2009).

The CAPE-V utilizes a 100-point visual-analog scale (VAS) for the perceptual qualities of overall severity, roughness, breathiness, strain, pitch, and loudness. The clinician makes a mark on a 100-mm line with the 0 point indicating no disturbance and the 100 mark indicating the maximum severity. The CAPE-V form is available on the American Speech-Language Hearing Association website (http://www.asha.org). The CAPE-V allows the clinician to add other perceptual parameters to the evaluation as well, such as glottal fry or hyper/hyponasality.

Documentation of the use of the CAPE-V with children has been reported for several clinical populations, including children with vocal fold nodules (e.g., Nuss, Ward, Huang, Volk, & Woodnorth, 2010) and children who are post-airway reconstruction and have residual upper airway and voice concerns (Kelchner et al., 2010). There are often methodological concerns about repeatability in perceptual analyses. Kelchner, Weinrich, Brehm, Tabangin, & de Alacron, (2010) found strong interreliability between expert raters for the parameters of breathiness, roughness, pitch, and overall severity. On the accompanying DVD, the reader can find samples of children saying sentences from the CAPE-V form and accompanying expert ratings.

As previously stated, the level of concern and the parents' perception of the voice disorder are essential to understand for the evaluating and treating clinicians. In two studies, the correlation between CAPE-V scores and pVHI scores for children with vocal fold nodules (Johnson, Brehm, Weinrich, Meinzen-Derr, & de Alarcon, 2011) and children who were post–airway reconstruction (de Alarcon et al., 2009) were evaluated. In both studies, the results revealed weak correlations between the clinician perception of the voice disorders and the parent perception. This is an important difference for clinicians to realize and highlights the need to truly understand the parent perspective for treatment planning.

Instrumental Assessment

The available instrumentation for evaluating laryngeal function has advanced substantially over the past 30 years. These advances allow for: (1) more precise diagnoses, (2) a better understanding of vocal function, and (3) an increased ability to predict recovery from a laryngeal disorder. Many of the evaluation techniques discussed in this section can be utilized as feedback tools during therapy.

The availability and diverse array of instruments to evaluate vocal function is increasing. Advances in technology in terms of size, affordability, and capability are rapid. Decisions related to choice of instrumentation and measurement selection can become an overwhelming task for the clinician. Choices may be limited by cost and availability, but ideally choices are made to fit specific patient populations. Another important concept to keep in mind when selecting instrumentation and measurements is that many commercially available products provide a large number of measures. It is the responsibility of the clinician to understand those measures and to report those that have clinical validity and that are most salient for the patient. As stated previously, at the end of this chapter, there are clinical setting scenarios that describe evaluation protocols tailored for specific patient settings.

Another challenge that clinicians face when incorporating instrumental measures in an evaluation is the lack of normative data on many of the key assessment variables. This problem exists to a greater degree in the realm of pediatric data versus adult data. As previously stated, a lack of correlation between auditory perceptual measures and instrumental evaluation measures has been cited in the literature (e.g., Shrivastav & Sapienza, 2003). Despite some of these concerns and some problems and pitfalls that will be mentioned for common measures in the upcoming sections, many of these measures can be used to monitor progress overtime in the treatment/therapy. Therefore, while sometimes the exact meaning of the magnitude of change in a measure may be poorly documented in the literature, the fact that the measure is changing over time may be helpful for motivating children/parents and for documentation purposes.

Although not discussed extensively in the literature, attention must be paid to the manner in which samples for analysis are obtained. This issue is not one that can be overlooked when assessing children. Types of cueing and methods for obtaining sounds may heavily impact the value of the measure. Examples of studies in which methods have differed or in which cues have been compared in children are discussed throughout this section of this chapter. As with all tasks that are utilized to describe physiologic aspects of speech and voice production, multiple trials (repeated measures) should be obtained. This concept, again, is essential to incorporate in the evaluation of children. Maximum performance tasks, such as maximum phonation time and maximum frequency range, are often unfamiliar novel tasks for children and they often exhibit a learning curve in performance.

Acoustic Analysis

There are many aspects of acoustic analysis of the voice that are attractive to the clinician working with children, including their noninvasive nature and the fact that they can be obtained fairly quickly. Another attractive feature of acoustic analysis is that much of the hardware/software components of signal capturing and analysis are in some cases becoming more affordable. Acoustic evaluation of voice is fast becoming accessible to more clinicians with the increased number of free downloadable recording/analysis software and apps. Some of the most common clinical acoustic measures obtained from children are fundamental frequency (F_0), intensity, perturbation, spectrography, and signal-to-noise ratio. This section will outline the procedures for obtaining these measures, as well as the many reliability and validity issues related to acoustic measures obtained from phonation with pathology that must be considered. A video example of a child completing an acoustic protocol can be found on the accompanying DVD.

Recording Considerations

There are many variables that can influence the outcome of an acoustic exam, including the recording procedures, environment, and instructions/methods, which are key for assessing children. Generally, the purpose of recording a signal is to obtain acoustic measures that pro-

vide more information about the underlying anatomy and physiology of the larynx. Additionally, acoustic recordings are made for later perceptual analysis, which also requires special attention to the quality of the recording methods. The typical components required for recording include a microphone, a preamplifier, and a recording device. Generally for speech/voice recordings, you would want the microphone to have a wide frequency response, a high sensitivity level, and a good signal-to-noise ratio. Fortunately, most commercially available recording devices have these features, which are appropriate for speech recording. In regard to recording software, sampling rate, which is essentially the number of digital "snapshots" the software takes of the inputted voice signal over time, should be at least 20 kHz. Clinicians should examine the settings in the software program they are using to find the default sampling rate, and change this as necessary.

Clinical Note: When purchasing a microphone, particularly for the first time for a clinical assessment setup, a clinician might choose to speak with a technician associated with the distributor to discuss the best and most economical choice.

Another potential problem to avoid during recording is peak clipping. Peak clipping is a phenomenon that can occur during recording when the intensity of the signal from a microphone is higher than the recording device/software is able to input. See Figure 5–1, which demonstrates an example of a peak-clipped and non–peak-clipped acoustic waveform. Special attention must be paid to internal input settings on computers as well as

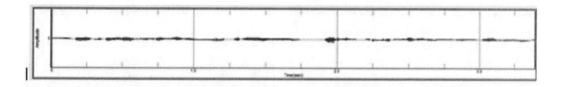

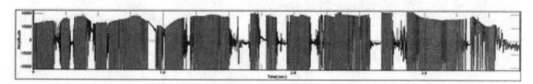

Figure 5–1. The top image shows a speech signal captured at a gain level that is too low. The bottom image shows a speech signal captured at a gain level that is too high. The signal is peak-clipped.

external controls on microphones and pream-plifiers. Peak clipping can be avoided by paying close attention to the gain, and clinicians need to be sure to record the gain setting and use the same setting for follow-up evaluations. While paying close attention to the gain, the clinician must be careful not to record a signal that is too low. Many commercially available software systems are unable to analyze and process a signal that does not have the minimum intensity required for the system.

> Clinical Note: Clinicians who evaluate children will encounter those who are shy or have almost aphonic voices, while others may have lesions and be loud or very boisterous. Gain settings may be required to change from patient to patient.

As previously mentioned, recordings should be in a sound-treated booth if possible, but certainly in a quiet room. Sounds with lower frequencies have longer wavelengths and tend to interfere with recordings from surrounding areas. This can be particu-

larly problematic, as these lower frequencies may overlap with the fundamental frequency of interest.

Instrumentation

The first consideration for acoustic measurement is the recording equipment utilized. The selection of equipment may be heavily based on the type of analyses the clinician wishes to perform and the use of the information. A fairly simple format of recording and analysis would be with a tablet/desktop/laptop built-in microphone and a pre-installed or downloadable recording/analysis software program such as Audacity or Wavesurfer. Recording requirements for research purposes are generally more stringent and require more than typical attention to the type of microphone, sound card quality, and recording software.

More sophisticated instrumentation setups are available from manufacturers such as KayPENTAX, which distributes acoustic analysis hardware/software setups ranging in regard to price and capability. Two common instrumentation setups are the Visi-Pitch IV (Model 3950) and the Computerized Speech Laboratory (Model 4500). These systems allow for recording of the acoustic signal as well as analysis of many of the common measures described in this section. An advantage of using these systems is the clear and often simplified (compared with some research tools available) screen display, which can demonstrate changes in pitch and loudness to patients. These systems are equipped with games and other biofeedback tools that can be used in therapy with children (see examples in Chapter 6).

Measures

Fundamental Frequency. Average fundamental frequency is defined as the average number of vibratory cycles of the vocal folds per second. Common measures of fundamental frequency include: (1) speaking fundamental frequency (SF_0), (2) frequency variability, and (3) frequency range. Data regarding frequency from several studies examining children utilizing different speech elicitation tasks are reported in Tables 5–3, 5–4, and 5–5.

SF_0 is typically extracted from a recorded sample of phrases or sentences, and its perceptual correlate is habitual pitch. Frequency has been found to covary with intensity due to laryngeal adjustments that are similar to increase both of these parameters. Therefore, it is important to document intensity levels used

Table 5–3. Mean Fundamental Frequency for Children 4:0 to 5:11 Years (*n* = 30 children)

Elicitation Task	Frequency (Hz)	Standard Error (SE)
Vowel	263.21	6.91
Counting	255.35	4.25
Storytelling	267.83	5.15

Source: Data from Brehm, Weinrich, Sprouse, May, & Hughes (2012).

Table 5–4. Fundamental Frequency Values in Children Age 5:0 to 7:11 Years (*n* = 48 children)

Elicitation Task	Frequency (Hz)	Standard Error (SE)	Range (Hz)
Vowel	240.46	2.96	182.87–294.07
Phrase	236.55	2.58	205.88–299.93
Sentence	235.66	2.97	172.96–294.99
Counting	246.51	2.76	212.48–300.83

Source: Data from Baker, Weinrich, Bevington, Schroth, & Shroeder (2008).

by a child during pre- and post-intervention assessments. Documenting gain and intensity levels is a point that is made frequently throughout this chapter. This concept is important when working with children who may be initially shy upon first meeting a clinician but then speak with more volume at a later point in time when there is an increased comfort level with the clinician and the types of tasks they are being asked to perform.

Maximum frequency phonation range (MFPR) is the range of frequencies that a child can produce. A healthy young adult should have approximately a three-octave range—a smaller range would be expected in children. MFPR is frequently used in evaluations, as improvements in range may indicate increased vocal flexibility and the potential resolution of vocal fold lesions that have previously added mass to the vocal folds. Frequency range tasks can be completed using several methodologies. The clinician might simply ask the child to glide up from a note at his or her mid-range to the highest note on a vowel or the word "whoop." Similarly, the clinician would ask the child to glide down

Table 5–5. Fundamental Frequency Values for Children Age 5 to 10 Years (*n* = 12)

Elicitation Task	Mean Frequency (Hz)	Standard Deviation (SD)	Range (Hz)
Count 1–10	215.21	16.40	195.26–247.83
Reading	228.45	23.53	196.97–284.30
Spontaneous Speech	224.31	24.78	181.56–281.07
Sustain /a/	224.59	22.93	186.11–272.61
Produce "um-hum"	226.19	20.08	188.35–259.83
Count 1–3 and sustain /i/	224.32	15.47	205.52–259.58
Produce "uh-huh"	214.64	10.12	200.27–229.34

Group composed of male and female children between age 5 and 10, with a mean of 8.3 years.
Source: Data from Zraick, Skaggs, & Montague (2000).

from a note at mid-range to his or her lowest note on a vowel or the word "boom." This methodology is generally referred to as a glissando task.

Perturbation. Perturbation is the short-term cycle-to-cycle variability observed in a speech signal. *Jitter* is the term used to describe the cycle-to-cycle variability observed in fundamental frequency. *Shimmer* is the term used to describe the cycle-to-cycle variability of intensity. Even healthy-appearing vocal folds will have variability that can be quantified; however, higher levels of variability are observed in patients with disorders of the larynx. An important point to remember when extracting these values with a clinical software program is that they should only be obtained from a sustained vowel, as connected speech would introduce large variability related to unvoiced and voiced sounds. It is important to note that many of the available clinical software programs will calculate these measures on a connected speech sample as it attempts to apply the measurement algorithm; however, the values reported are meaningless.

There are several drawbacks to the use of short-term variability measures in children.

There is a significant lack of normative data for these measures, and therefore interpreting the significance of values or defining a disordered from a nondisordered voice is not possible. Additionally there is a lack of documentation in the literature that these measures correlate with deficits in perceptual qualities (Wolfe, Fitch, & Martin, 1997). Likely the most significant limitation in the use of this measure is that it can only be extracted from voice signals that have a reliable and identifiable fundamental frequency. Identifying a reliable fundamental frequency signal is discussed further in the "Sound Spectrography" section. Despite some of these drawbacks, these measures can be used to monitor patient progress, as they can show change with improvement in laryngeal health and function; however, the magnitude of change may not be known.

Intensity. Vocal intensity is defined as the acoustic power of the sound produced by the child. *Intensity* is generally used as the term of the measurable component, and *loudness* is used as the descriptive or perceptual correlate. There is not a linear relationship between measured intensity values and the perception of loudness. The most commonly reported measure of intensity is average intensity. In children, particularly those who have significant laryngeal scarring or mobility issues, the inability to produce a louder voice when desired is a significant voice complaint. In these children, it may also be useful to measure maximum intensity. These measures can be obtained from connected speech or during the sustaining of a vowel sound.

Many acoustical software measurement packages have the ability to produce a measurement of intensity. There are several factors that must be understood and controlled for when obtaining intensity measures with these programs. Importantly, many of these software programs report intensity, in decibels (dB) relative to an internal reference value. This is not a measure of decibel sound pressure level (dB SPL), but rather a relative value. Therefore, intensity values obtained from the same child in terms of pre/posttherapy or surgical evaluations from the same instrumentation have the capability of showing a measureable change in intensity (reported in dB). Caution should be used in interpreting change in intensity values if the same software/analysis package is not used to obtain the measures pre- and posttreatment.

There are several factors that must be controlled when obtaining measurements of intensity. All attempts must be made to reduce or eliminate ambient noise. If possible, measures can be obtained in a sound-treated booth. Ambient noise can be of particular concern in a school setting in which the SLP's office may be located next to classrooms, gymnasiums, and/or cafeterias. Another important factor that must be controlled is mouth-to-microphone distance. Again, this factor can be challenging with children, as they are more likely to move about during the assessment. For some children, using a head-worn microphone in which the distance can be easily held constant may be of benefit. Consistent mouth-to-microphone distance and control of input gain level are key when making assessments of progress and change in regard to intensity over time.

If a clinician is not able to use a software program for the measurement of intensity, a hand-held sound level meter such as one sold by RadioShack may be used. The range of intensity that can be measured by a meter such as this is 50 to 126 dB SPL. Additionally, there are a variety of settings that the clinician can adjust (e.g., weighting filters, fast/slow response). When used in an evaluation with a child, the clinician could hold the device a certain distance from the child's mouth (commonly 50 cm) and report an average dB SPL value viewed on the display screen. The clinician should be sure to record the distance from the mouth utilized in the examination for comparison of future recordings.

Signal/Harmonic-to-Noise Ratio. Signal-to-noise ratio (SNR) and harmonic-to-noise ratio (HNR) are synonymous terms. Both refer to a measurement that is a ratio of the energy from the fundamental frequency to the energy found in the noise or aperiodic component of the voice. Potential sources of "noise" during phonation include excessive air escape during the closed phase of vibration due to vocal fold weakness or paralysis. There are other causes of short-term variation in vocal fold vibration, such as fatigue and excessive mucus, which make the reliability/repeatability of these measures problematic for some patients (i.e., children with otherwise healthy vocal folds may demonstrate abnormal values due to short-term issues). The algorithms used to measure SNR from clinical software programs vary so much that it is actually difficult to compare values obtained from different systems. Therefore, reporting normative values for this measure is challenging as well as likely misleading. Many software programs include normative values for their particular system.

Under the appropriate conditions, this measure can be meaningful for comparison of voice production in a child over time. As with many of the previous measures discussed, SNR can only be obtained from a voice signal in which the F_0 must be identifiable.

Voice Range Profile

The voice range profile (VRP) is an evaluation method that examines the range of frequencies and intensities that a child can produce. This evaluation method would typically be reserved for a child who has a significant interest in singing and is reporting difficulty in the singing voice.

Sound Spectrography

Sound spectrography is a graphic display of a sound in terms of its frequency and intensity over time. This graphic display is called a spectrogram. On a spectrogram, frequency is displayed on the *y*-axis, time is displayed on the *x*-axis, and intensity is displayed by different levels of darkness (the darker the line, the more intense; Figure 5–2). In Figure 5–2, one can observe the F_0, which is the lowest energy band. All of the bands above this are harmonics and those that represent resonating frequencies for that sound have the most amplitude (intensity) and are called formant frequencies. There are two types of spectrograms: wideband and narrowband. Wideband spectrograms offer better time resolution but less frequency resolution, and thus fewer harmonics can be clearly viewed. Narrowband spectrograms, on the other hand, have poorer time resolution but better frequency resolution and therefore all harmonics and noise in between them is clearly displayed. This clear display of harmonics and noise is essential for evaluating voice signal types (Titze, 1994). Using this type of spectrogram, a signal can be classified into one of three types. When a voice signal has clearly defined harmonics without bands of noise that appear (light-colored horizontal lines) between those harmonics, it is identified as a *type 1* voice signal. When significant bands/horizontal lines appear between the harmonics, these are identified as "subharmonics" and the voice is classified as a *type II* signal. There are some voice signals in which there is no clearly identifiable harmonic structure. Those signals are classified as *type III* signals. Examples of these signal types are displayed in Figure 5–3.

As you can see, analysis of a spectrogram is an excellent starting point for analyzing acoustic signals from children. It is important to note that despite issues regarding the validity of measures from sound signals that do not have identifiable F_0 or have much noise and banding between the harmonics, most clinical software programs will compute all of the potential measures from the program.

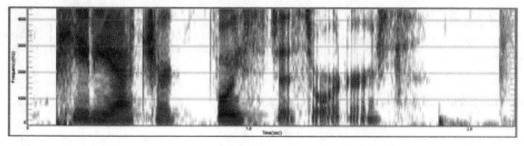

Figure 5–2. The phrase "Pediatric Voice Disorders" is displayed as a wideband spectrogram.

Type 1

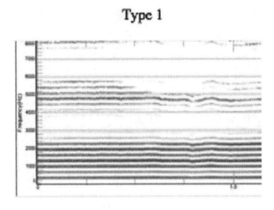

Type 2

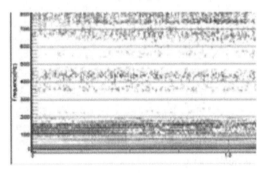

Type 3

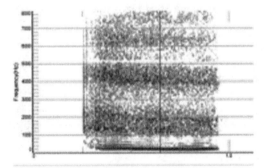

Figure 5–3. All three images are narrow-band spectrograms displaying acoustic signal types.

It is essential for the evaluating clinician to determine whether or not those measures are accurate.

A second type of display of a sound is completed by doing a Fourier analysis or a breakdown of a sound at a moment in time into all of its frequency components. The display result is called a line spectrum or a spectral analysis. On this display, the *y*-axis represents amplitude and the *x*-axis represents frequency.

The limitations posed by the inability to extract some acoustic measures from voice samples of patients with dysphonia have prompted the exploration of other measures that might differentiate healthy from disordered voices. One such examination with children (Meredith et al., 2008) provided the first report of nonlinear dynamic measures in children with dysphonia. The nonlinear dynamic parameter of correlation (D_2) and jitter percent were both found to be statistically different between children with dysphonia and children with normal voice. However, larger standard deviations and *p*-values were observed in the comparison of jitter, indicating that this parameter may be less reliable than the D_2 parameter.

Analysis of Dysphonia in Speech and Voice

The Analysis of Dysphonia in Speech and Voice (ADSV™) (KayPENTAX) is a new software that uses cepstral/spectral analysis to provide objective estimates of dysphonia for both sustained voice and continuous speech samples (Figure 5–4; Awan & Roy, 2009). Measures of cepstral/spectral index of dysphonia (CSID) have been shown to correlate well with expert perceptual evaluations of disordered voices in global ratings of dysphonia (Awan, Roy, & Dromey, 2009; Awan, Roy, Jette, Meltzner, & Hillman, 2010). To generate the CSID, the ADSV requires separate analysis of each sentence on the CAPE-V. Therefore, different CSID estimates can be obtained for the different sentence types (e.g., all voiced, easy onset). Using ADSV it is possible to examine the relationship between the specific parameters of voice, sentence type,

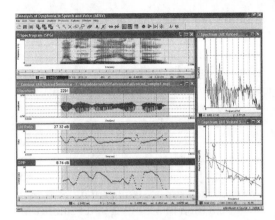

Figure 5–4. Screenshot of Analysis of Dysphonia in Speech and Voice (ADSV) software. Courtesy of KayPENTAX.

and the CSID. Thus, the ADSV overcomes some of the limitations of traditional acoustic assessment, particularly when assessing severely disordered voices in children.

Aerodynamics

Measures of laryngeal aerodynamics examine the airflow and pressures that are produced during speech production. Importance is placed on the examination of these characteristics during voicing, as they are assumed to play a large role in vocal fold oscillation. Obtaining aerodynamic measures is becoming more common for voice evaluation teams and many private-practice clinicians. Increased marketing of instrumentation setups and orientation of these setups toward the practicing clinician (as opposed to using these values primarily in research) is likely the cause for the increased use. Aerodynamic measures are considered to be noninvasive and include measurements of airflow, pressure, and resistance within the vocal tract as well as duration measures (e.g., maximum phonation time). A video example of a child being prepared for

an aerodynamic assessment can be found on the accompanying DVD.

Instrumentation

There are several clinical instrumentation packages available for the evaluation of aerodynamic measures. The main component of each of these setups is a pneumotachograph. A pneumotachograph is an instrument that has a means of sensing pressure differentials during airflow. The pneumotach pictured in Figure 5–5 is a traditional flow head. Contained within this pneumotach are two metal mesh screens through which airflow passes. There are pressure sensors connected to these screens that detect the pressure differential or drop in pressure as it passes through these screens. Average airflow rate is derived from this drop in pressure. Generally during the evaluation of a voice disorder, these signals are obtained from a sustained vowel rather than connected speech.

Another commonly used pneumotachograph in the area of speech and voice measurement is a Rothenberg circumferentially vented pneumotachograph (Figure 5–6). The

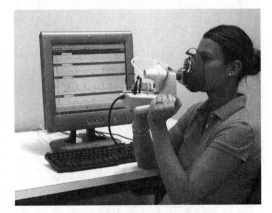

Figure 5–5. Traditional flowhead pneumotachograph (KayPENTAX Phonatory Aerodynamic System (PAS). Courtesy of KayPENTAX.

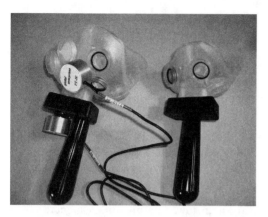

Figure 5–6. Photo courtesy of Glottal Enterprises, Syracuse, NY. At left: large (adult/teen-size) mask, with the pressure transducer sensing airflow mounted in one of the holes in the mask wall provided for this purpose. At right: a small (small size) mask with the pressure transducer mounted within the mask handle, as used by Glottal Enterprises for measuring nasal emission in their Nasality Visualization System, or for measuring oral consonant airflow in their Consonant Visualization System. Reproduced with permission from Glottal Enterprises, Syracuse, NY.

tributor has sizes that are appropriate for even small children. All of the setups have a means of calibrating the instrumentation as well. Generally, calibration of aerodynamic equipment requires a means of introducing a known airflow volume or rate into the pneumotachograph.

There have been several criticisms regarding the alteration of breathing patterns provided by wearing a mask during speech; however, there are no significant differences in documentation of breathing and volume during speech production demonstrated during mask-on and mask-off conditions in young women (using a circumferentially vented mask; Huber, Stathopoulos, Bormann, & Johnson, 1998). Children, particularly those who have undergone multiple previous surgeries, may associate a face mask with receiving anesthesia. It is important to know that some children may be afraid of the mask at first and may benefit from activities such as touching the mask (carefully!) and smelling the mask while being reassured that it is going to be used to obtain information about their speech—not put them to sleep.

structure of this mask allows for more preservation of vowel qualities by minimizing sound distortion and preventing the loss of high frequencies. This mask was developed by Martin Rothenberg. The pressure differential in this mask is measured by the impedance imposed by a wire cloth screen made of fine mesh steel embedded within the mask itself. The ability to preserve vowel qualities allows for more sophisticated or finely detailed aerodynamic measures, which are described below in the section on "Inverse Filtering." Currently this is the only type of mask that can be used to obtain the timing and speed measures described in that section.

All of the available instrumentation setups have a mask that provides a tight seal to the face. Generally the commercial dis-

Measures

Several commonly obtained aerodynamic measures are described in the following sections. Multiple studies are available in the literature in which values for these measures are provided for children, and references for some of these studies are provided. Recently, a study obtaining normative values on a variety of normative measures in 60 children age 6 to 18 years was published, and some of the relevant measures to the discussion below are reported in Table 5–6.

Estimated Subglottal Pressure. The pressure generated by the lungs during speech production is a common parameter evaluated in patients with voice disorders. This measure

Table 5–6. Normative Aerodynamic Data in Children Age 6:0 to 17:11 Years

Gender	6:0–9:11 years (n = 20)		10:0–13:11 years (n = 20)		14–17:11 years (n = 20)	
	Mean (SD)	Range	Mean (SD)	Range	Mean (SD)	Range
Female						
Maximum Phonation time (s)	11.30 (2.36)	8.16–14.68	19.40 (6.95)	13.02–35.77	23.12 (5.09)	15.11–29.56
Mean expiratory airflow (L/s)	0.14 (0.05)	0.07–0.23	0.14 (0.04)	0.06–0.22	0.15 (0.03)	0.11–0.22
Mean peak air pressure (cm H_2O)	10.08 (2.59)	5.59–13.31	9.12 (3.01)	6.12–15.86	8.14 (2.75)	4.85–13.45
Aerodynamic resistance ([cm H_2O]/[L/s])	92.77 (47.22)	50.81–168.58	62.69 (29.13)	29.84–131.10	46.67 (10.23)	29.79–61.93
Male						
Maximum Phonation time (s)	12.51 (2.85)	7.24–16.38	16.47 (4.60)	6.42–24.29	22.37 (7.20)	9.34–34.45
Mean expiratory airflow (L/s)	0.17 (0.10)	0.09–0.43	0.17 (0.06)	0.10–0.28	0.23 (0.15)	0.07–0.54
Mean peak air pressure (cm H_2O)	10.90 (2.98)	6.66–15.47	9.66 (2.69)	6.13–14.58	8.40 (2.27)	6.07–12.32
Aerodynamic resistance ([cm H_2O]/[L/s])	75.06 (30.78)	33.16–116.80	52.15 (17.51)	28.08–80.89	40.49 (17.53)	19.46–72.65

Source: Data from Weinrich, Brehm, Knudsen, McBride, & Hughes (2012).

is commonly referred to as *estimated subglottal pressure*. Generally, larger than expected pressure values compared with normative values indicate an element of hyperfunction of the laryngeal mechanism. Estimated subglottal pressure is the pressure directly beneath the vocal folds during voicing. The term "estimated" is used during most clinical evaluations, as this measure is obtained indirectly from pressures measured in the oral cavity. The only means of directly measuring this value are through tracheal puncture or through a tracheostomy tube. For estimated subglottal pressure, the specific pressure that is measured is in the oral cavity during the closed portion of a voiceless bilabial consonant (/p/) that immediately follows a vowel. The pressure is detected with the use of a polyethylene tube between the lips connected to a transducer. The task that is generally performed is a syllable train of /pa-pa. . . ./ or /pi-pi. . ./. The recommended rate for the syllable train production is 1.5 syllables per second. The measures can be obtained accurately at a slightly slower rate, but a faster rate than 1.5 syllables per second would not allow the pressure to equalize in the upper respiratory tract. The repetition of the syllable seven times in a row is a common recommendation with adults. This number of repetitions can be very difficult for some children, but the goal should be to have at least five repetitions. Generally, the middle 3 to 5 syllables are used for measurement. Children should be reminded not to chew or bite on the tube or obstruct it with the tongue.

Laryngeal Airflow. Laryngeal airflow is the volume of air that passes through the glottis during a set period of time. It is important to remember that this measure is a gross estimate of function, as the airflow through the upper respiratory tract is influenced not only by the valving characteristics of the larynx, but also by the vocal tract structures that modulate the airflow. The influence of other airway structures on average airflow rates limits its use as a *fine, discrete* measurement of laryngeal function. Average airflow rates are typically reported in milliliters per second and are obtained from sustaining a vowel. Values for average airflow vary greatly. Research with both children and adults reveal that the use of a breathy voice or a hypofunctioning larynx produces higher airflow rates, whereas use of a pressed voice or a hyperfunctioning larynx increases airflow rates. Average airflow rate values observed from several studies examining aerodynamic measures in children are found in Table 5–6.

Laryngeal Resistance. The methodology for obtaining laryngeal resistance was introduced by Smitheran and Hixon (1981). Laryngeal resistance is the impedance of the airway during voice production by the valving of the glottis. This measure is calculated as a ratio of estimated subglottal pressure over average airflow.

Inverse Filtering. Inverse filtering is a procedure that essentially removes the contribution of the vocal tract. The waveform that results following inverse filtering is a representation of the airflow at the level of the vocal folds or glottis. Many of the measures obtained from this waveform examine open and closure timing and speed characteristics. Common measures from the glottal airflow waveform observed in the literature include: open quotient, maximum flow declination rate (MFDR), peak glottal airflow, alternating glottal airflow, and minimum glottal airflow. Values from these measures in children are reported to a limited extent in the literature. Weinrich, Salz, and Hughes (2005) completed a normative data study examining the glottal airflow waveform in 75 children ages 6 to 10 years. Stathopoulos and Sapienza (1997) completed a developmental examination of these measures in children ages 4 to

14 years. Values obtained from inverse filtered aerodynamic signals have also been reported for children with vocal fold nodules (Sapienza & Stathopoulos, 1994).

Maximum Phonation Time. Maximum phonation time (MPT) is frequently included in voice assessments with children. It is an "easy" measure to obtain, requiring little instrumentation, and is commonly used when no formal aerodynamic instrumentation is available. MPT is obtained by asking the child to sustain a vowel at a comfortable pitch and loudness level for as long as he or she possibly can. This measurement can easily be obtained by using a stopwatch. Many speech recording/analysis software programs can also be used to measure the time of phonation as well as provide visual feedback to the child while performing the task. The reliability of this measure relies on the child inspiring to total lung capacity and breathing out to residual volume. This task, particularly with young children, requires modeling and verbal encouragement. The reliability and validity of this measure has been greatly called into question throughout the literature, indicating that a large number of trials is required for consistency in children (e.g., Finnegan, 1984). Completion of a large number of trials can be problematic from an attention and fatigue standpoint. However, when utilizing this measure it is recommended that at least three trials be obtained. Not utilizing significant proportions of vital capacity for this task has been documented in adults as well (Solomon, Garlitz, & Milbrath, 2000). It is important to understand the criticisms of a measure such as MPT and to use this measure only in combination with other physiologic measures that describe vocal and respiratory function.

s/z Ratio. The s/z ratio is a quick screening method that may provide some information about abnormal airflow in the presence of a vocal fold lesion. To obtain this ratio, the clinician asks the child to sustain /s/ for as long as possible. Subsequently, the child is asked to sustain /z/ for as long as possible. Verbal encouragement throughout the tasks is highly recommended, and the use of biofeedback on a digital/software recording program (on a computer) may be helpful as well with young children. As with all maximum performance evaluations, practice and demonstration as well as the averaging of multiple trials (at least three) are important. The adult literature generally points to the acceptance of a 1.0 ratio comparing the /s/ with the /z/ as an indication of a healthy voice. A recent large-scale normative study of children indicated that most healthy children had a ratio close to 1.0 (Tavares, Brasolotto, Rodrigues, Benito Pessin, & Garcia Martins, 2012). If the /s/ is much longer than the /z/, this discrepancy could indicate glottal closure incompetence/insufficiency due to an abnormality of the vocal folds. Due to the maximal performance nature of these tasks, all of the concerns discussed above related to MPT apply to this measure. Therefore, again this measure should never be used in isolation to describe vocal function.

Electroglottography

Electroglottography (EGG) is a method of evaluation that examines the vocal fold contact area patterns during vibration. The technology is considered to be noninvasive, with electrodes being placed just on the surface of the skin on either side of the thyroid cartilage. A very small, low-voltage current passes through the electrodes when vocal fold contact is made. The benefit of EGG analysis with children is that it is noninvasive. In fact, Cheyne, Nuss, and Hillman (1999) completed a normative data study of EGG measures in children and found that children as young as 3 years tolerated the procedure well. Additional studies have reported successful use of EGG in children as young as 7 years (e.g., Linders, Massa, Boersma, & Dejonckere, 1995; Pedersen, Moller, Krabbe, Bennett, & Svenstrup, 1990).

Endoscopic

A variety of evaluation tools are utilized for endoscopic examination of the larynx in a child with a voice disorder. Dynamic digital (formerly video) laryngeal stroboscopic imaging, which provides a simulated slow motion view of vocal fold vibration, has been the gold standard examination of voice for over 25 years (Bless, Hirano, & Feder, 1987). The rate of human vocal fold vibration is typically in the average F_0 range of 110 to 400 Hz (depending on age and gender), which is too fast for the human eye to see. Digital endostroboscopy involves the use of a rigid endoscope (Figure 5–7) presented transorally and positioned above the child's larynx. The 70° angle lens directs the light into the larynx as the child sustains the sound "ee." The magnified image is viewed on the computer screen, where the examiner can make important observations about laryngeal function and vocal fold vibration. The vibratory parameters viewed in this exam are dependent on the acoustic (voice) signal, which is tracked via a stethoscope microphone placed at the neck. The acoustic signal triggers the stroboscopic light, which flashes slightly out of phase (slower) with the F_0. Each flash captures a point across successive cycles of vibration, and the image is fused to recreate a representative glottic vibratory cycle (Figures 5–8 and 5–9). This imaging technique relies heavily on periodicity (regularity) of the acoustic signal to create an accurate image of vibratory motion; however, the population of individuals with voice disorders often presents with irregular and aperiodic voice signals (type II or III).

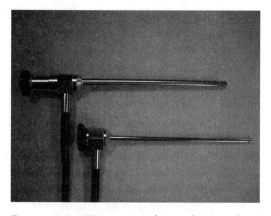

Figure 5–7. This image shows the standard size rigid scope on top and a pediatric rigid scope with a smaller diameter on the bottom. Courtesy of KayPENTAX.

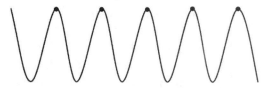

Figure 5–8. Still image will result when the stroboscopic light is pulsed at exactly the same frequency as the fundamental frequency.

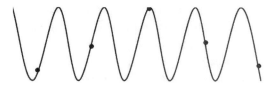

Figure 5–9. A simulated slow motion image will occur when the stroboscopic light is pulsed at a slightly slower frequency than the fundamental frequency

Two types of clinical ratings are made from these images: gross laryngeal and discrete vibratory. It is the discrete vibratory motions (mucosal wave, amplitude of vibration, glottal closure, periodicity, phase symmetry) that can be lost or distorted if the signal has significant frequency perturbations. Interpreting stroboscopic images requires careful training and continuous calibration with other endostroboscopists. On the accompanying DVD the reader can find samples of pediatric strobe exams and accompanying expert ratings. Given the differences in pediatric vocal fold microstructure, interpretation of simulated slow motion images of vibratory motion might yield differences when compared with those of adults. At this time any such differences have not been described. A sample of explaining an endoscopic examination to a child can be found on the accompanying DVD.

The selection of the evaluation instrument is often based on the availability of equipment, the age of the child, and the cooperation of the child. Rigid endoscopy can be performed with cooperative children ages 6 and above (Hartnick & Zeitels, 2005), but anecdotal clinical reports suggest that brief views can be captured in very cooperative children as young as 3 years of age. The ability to view the vocal folds with rigid endoscopy in young children may prevent some direct laryngeal examinations under anesthesia. Older children tolerate a standard adult rigid scope; however, a smaller Hopkins rod pediatric rigid scope is available (see Figure 5–7). Pediatric fiberoptic endoscopes are available that have a smaller diameter (2.2 to 2.4 mm), which is often suitable for children under the age of 4 years. Although a smaller scope may be required for cooperation of the child, the image quality is lower compared with images obtained with larger diameter scopes. Pediatric chip-in-the-tip scopes (3.2 mm in diameter) provide much higher image quality and can be used with most children over the age of 4 years (Figure 5–10). Any child undergoing a flexible fiberoptic or distal chip examination will receive some type of topical anesthetic and nasal decongestant to minimize discomfort unless it is contraindicated. This medication is applied by a nurse or physician. Of

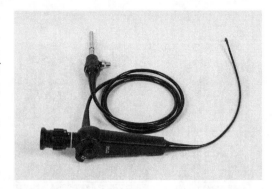

Figure 5–10. KayPENTAX flexible fiberoptic endoscopes: 10R3P version 2. Courtesy of KayPENTAX.

equal importance is the preparation for the exam in order to inform the parent and child about what is involved in the exam protocol. Often the SLP leads this discussion.

Using the same endoscopic techniques to obtain a stroboscopic image, high-speed imaging technology is now available to record actual cycle-by-cycle vibration. Using commercial systems, images are captured at 2,000 to 4,000 frames per second (fps) and are viewed using slow-motion playback (30 fps). Images can be captured using black and white or color cameras depending on the needed frame rate (Figure 5–11). Frame rates for recording depend on the F_0 of the signal (participant's voice). Color recordings are clear only up to 3,000 fps (KayPENTAX, 2011), and signals higher than that should be captured in black and white. Because of the large amount of data, only a maximum of 4 seconds can be recorded per exam. Ratings specific to high speed include: phase symmetry (anterior-posterior, left to right), open quotient (the time associated with the opening and closing phase of the vibratory cycle versus the duration of the entire vibratory cycle), cycle to cycle voice onset/offset (observation of whether contact and loss of contact change from cycle to cycle), glottic closure, and regularity or periodicity of the vibratory cycle (the exact

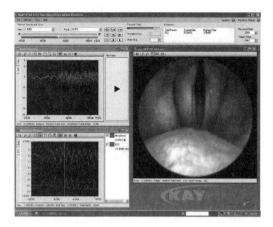

Figure 5–11. Screenshot of high-speed imaging. Courtesy of KayPENTAX.

repetition of a spatiotemporal pattern). Measures related to vocal attack time, frequency of vibration, rapid laryngeal maneuvers (crying, coughing, etc.), and kymography (see a description of this technology in the following section) can also be made, at a later time.

Either rigid or flexible endoscopes can be used to obtain the images, but at this time the flexible endoscopes used for high-speed imaging use a black and white camera. A major benefit of this technology is that assessment of signals with irregularities or aperiodicity no longer presents a problem. High-speed images of vibration can be analyzed for healthy and disordered vocal folds yielding new insights into fundamental vibratory mechanics and the effect of disease states, healing, and high performance use (e.g., trained singers).

Other vibratory events and laryngeal activity can also be captured via high-speed technology for subsequent analyses. For example, in the case of the post–airway reconstruction patient, it is not unusual to observe structures other than the true vocal folds vibrating. There is documentation of various distinct vibratory sources (Kelchner, Weinrich, et al., 2010) in numerous children who

have undergone reconstruction, but to date clinicians have been unable to further characterize the exact vibratory characteristics. This is especially important data to analyze in this population, as voice quality can be significantly altered by the initial laryngeal injury and subsequent surgical procedures. Understanding how an individual can generate voice and what types of vibratory activity are associated with various voice qualities will inform surgical, medical, and behavioral treatments.

Kymography technology has been available since the 1990s (Schutte, Svec, & Sram, 1998) and is used primarily for research purposes, although it does have specific clinical applications. There are actually three versions of this technology: videokymography (VKM), high-speed digital kymography (DKG), and strobovideokymography (SVKG; Švec and Schutte, 2012). VKM uses images captured at a very high rate (e.g., 8,000 fps) from a single line along the vocal fold in real time and as such can overcome the issue of signal perturbation. The successive cycles of vibration representing a point along the vocal fold are then displayed via a kymogram that is produced immediately (Plate 10). In this way discrete vibratory motion for that position can be analyzed.

DKG requires use of a digital high-speed system and kymographic software (Švec and Schutte, 2012) so kymographic images are developed later after processing. Discrete observations of vibratory behavior can be observed, but some limitations exist due to the large amount of storage required by capturing high-speed images. Mulitple kymograms can be generated. As with VKG, DKG overcomes issues related to vibratory irregularities, permitting a more discrete analysis of abnormal vibratory behavior. SVKG yields kymograms developed from standard stroboscopic exams and as such depends on a stable pitch for accurate image capture and interpretation. There are no limits to the amount of data captured.

There are numerous discrete phonatory parameters that can be rated using kymography, including voice onset and offset, mucosal wave, amplitude of vibration, phase symmetry, phase closure and periodicity, and discrete observations of right and left vocal fold edge vibratory abnormalities. Selecting the representative position or line along the vocal fold edge is determined by the goal of the exam. Importantly, VKM can be used to analyze the vibratory behavior of other tissue, such as the ventricular folds (Hertegård, 2005).

Given the large amount of vibratory data gathered, selecting the representative successive cycles of vibration for analysis can be daunting. Automated analysis of various vocal fold features, vibratory characteristics, and minimum capture rates, in frames per second, was described by Deliyski et al. (2008) and Deliyski and Hillman (2010). The reader is referred to those articles and work by Jan Švec and Harm Schutte for comprehensive information on this important technology and its application in furthering our knowledge about normal and abnormal vocal fold vibration.

Pulling It All Together: Case Summaries

The following section describes an evaluation format that could be followed in three different evaluation settings. The setting is described in terms of location, personnel, and equipment availability. This case example format is used to illustrate expected values, common scenarios, and challenges faced in specific settings with different types of disorders. Decisions regarding evaluation procedures are discussed based on the location and the case example patient.

Case 1. Hospital-Based Clinician

A 4-year-old female presented with vocal fold paralysis to a major metropolitan hospital equipped with a voice care team. The parents of the child initially queried the child's pediatrician about her voice quality, which had been hoarse since birth. The pediatrician made a referral for a voice evaluation to the geographically closest hospital with a voice care team. The following are the components of the evaluation that were utilized and sample results.

Case History

The clinician utilized a standard medical history form that the parents completed prior to the visit. The parents reported that the child was premature (29 weeks) and had required assistance with breathing at birth. She was intubated for 1 week. While addressing all aspects of the medical history form, the clinician spent the majority of the time during the child/parent interview asking questions about the number and length of intubations and whether the child was ever trached or had any feeding or swallowing difficulties.

Voice Quality of Life

The clinician chose to have the parents complete the Pediatric Voice Handicap Index (pVHI). The scores on this tool were as follows: Physical = 25; Emotional = 17; Functional = 22; Total = 64. These findings helped the clinician understand that the child/parents were somewhat limited socially by the dysphonia, but the physical limitations were the primary concern.

Acoustic Analysis

This child presented with a quiet and breathy voice. She was initially very shy during the recording segments for the acoustic and perceptual analysis. Due to her low volume, the clinician adjusted (raised) the gain on the preamplifier that was connected to the microphone and computer. The clinician made a note of the change in setting in the child's documentation for future reference. Due to the significant breathy component of the voice, the clinician initially had the child sustain /a/ and examined the narrowband spectrogram of this vowel. The spectrogram revealed that the voice signal had some identifiable harmonics but extensive noise-banding between them. Her voice was labeled as type II, thus significantly reducing the acoustic measures obtained during the exam (see discussion of signal typing in the "Sound Spectrography" section). The clinician did obtain an average intensity value, which was 68 dB, using the Computerized Speech Laboratory (Model 4500; KayPENTAX).

Aerodynamic Analysis

The clinician utilized the Phonatory Aerodynamic System (KayPENTAX) for the aerodynamic analysis. The child appeared to be initially apprehensive about putting a mask over her mouth; therefore, the clinician allowed her to touch the mask and showed her that she was able to breathe and talk with ease while the mask was in place. The child was able to complete a sustained vowel for average airflow measurement for about 5 seconds but required extensive instruction and modeling to complete the /pa-pa-pa. . ./ syllable train for the measurement of estimated subglottal pressure. After practice and models, she was able to provide a sample of five connected /pa/ syllables (the middle three syllables were used for the measurement). Her average airflow rate was 350 mL/s and her estimated subglottal pressure was 9 cm H_2O. The high rate of airflow is consistent with her vocal fold paralysis and glottal incompetence. Because the clinician had access to an aerodynamic

measurement system, she did not choose to complete other potential measures such as s/z ratio.

Laryngostroboscopic Evaluation

An attempt was made to complete a rigid endoscopic examination of the child using a pediatric scope (KayPENTAX 9018). Despite coaching and assistance with position, it was very difficult to view the full length of the child's vocal fold during the rigid examination. Additionally the child had a fairly omega-shaped epiglottis that limited the view of the vocal folds. An appropriate view of the vocal fold anatomy and laryngeal function was obtained using a flexible endoscope. The child poorly tolerated the chip-in-the-tip camera because of narrow nares, and therefore a fiberoptic camera was used. The endoscopic evaluation revealed immobility of the left vocal fold, paralyzed in a paramedian position. All other structures of the larynx appeared to be normal and healthy. There was no hyperfunction of supraglottic structures.

Perceptual Analysis

Following the evaluation, the clinician completed a perceptual analysis of the child's voice using the CAPE-V tool. The results of the analysis revealed the following scores: Overall Severity = 74; Roughness = 20; Breathiness = 72; Pitch = cannot rate; Loudness = 68. Her high breathiness score was consistent with her vocal fold paralysis, and the high loudness score (soft intensity) was consistent with one of the parents' primary complaints that she had difficulty making her voice louder.

Case 2. School-Based Clinician

A 10-year-old male with vocal nodules was identified as having a hoarse voice by his classroom teacher. The teacher referred the child to the school SLP. The child was then seen by a local otolaryngologist who completed a flexible laryngoscopic examination in the office through an eyepiece and diagnosed the child with bilateral vocal fold nodules. The otolaryngologist recommended a course of voice therapy. The school SLP had a written report about the laryngeal findings from the otolaryngologist.

Case History

The clinician utilized a medical history form that was completed by the child's parents. The parents reported that the child had been hoarse for many years; in fact, they could not identify when the hoarseness began. The child was involved in many extracurricular activities, including soccer, basketball, and baseball. The parents reported that the child frequently lost his voice following games in which he cheered and yelled a lot. A discussion with the child's classroom teacher revealed that he sometimes lost his voice following recess activities or gym class.

pVHI

The clinician mailed a pVHI form to the child's parents to complete. The scores on this tool were as follows: Physical = 26; Emotional = 11; Functional = 9; Total = 46. These findings helped the clinician understand that the child/parents were not limited socially by the dysphonia, but the physical limitations were the primary concern.

Acoustic Analysis

The clinician evaluating the child utilized a laptop computer with a microphone and preamplifier for recording. She had a prepackaged software program installed on her computer that allowed her to complete recordings and analysis parameters such as F_0, SF_0, jitter, shimmer, SNR, etc. She recorded a series of voice samples from the child and later examined a narrowband spectrogram of a sustained vowel. The clinician judged the voice signal to be type I. Therefore, the clinician felt confident regarding the accuracy of the fundamental frequency measures obtained. The child's SF_0 was 234 Hz, which was judged to be at the lower end of frequencies observed in children his age.

Aerodynamic Analysis

The clinician did not have an aerodynamic assessment system; however, she completed a gross evaluation of laryngeal airflow modification by having the child perform both the MPT and s/z ratio tasks. The child's MPT was 6 seconds and his s/z ratio was 1.3. The results of this analysis revealed excessive air may have been escaping due to incomplete closure of the glottis. It is important to remember that these measures are subject to many factors (as described previously in this chapter), should be used primarily as screening tools, and in this case could have been used as a means of documenting progress (but always in conjunction with other measures).

Perceptual Analysis

Following the evaluation, the clinician completed a perceptual analysis of the child's voice using the CAPE-V tool while listening to recordings of the child's voice. The results of the analysis revealed the following scores: Overall Severity = 14; Roughness = 12; Breathiness = 10; Pitch (low) = 15; Loudness (loud) = 17. The clinician also noted that most of her scores indicated that perceptually the voice was very mildly dysphonic. Based on the case history of this patient, the results of a perceptual analysis might be markedly different after heavy voice use from this child.

Case 3. Private Practice Clinician

Case history

This patient was a 14-year-old male with puberphonia referred from a hospital-based voice care team approximately 100 miles from the clinician's office. The team sent a DVD with the recorded examination in which a flexible endoscopic examination revealed healthy and normal-appearing laryngeal structures. However, throughout the voicing tasks performed during the examination, laryngeal tension was obvious and poor vocal fold closure was observed. The written report from the team indicated a diagnosis of puberphonia.

pVHI

The clinician gave a copy of the pVHI form to the child's parents but encouraged the child to participate in the completion of the form due to his age. The scores on this tool were as follows: Physical = 21; Emotional = 28; Functional = 14; Total = 63. These findings helped the clinician understand the large emotional impact of the voice problem for the child at this point in time.

Acoustic Analysis

The clinician focused on documenting several key acoustic measures during the evaluation, including SF_0 and intensity. During sentence production, the child's SF_0 was 290 Hz and average intensity was 69 dB. The results indicate that his SF_0 was in the higher range of normal for his age and his intensity was reduced.

Aerodynamic Analysis

The clinician did not have access to an aerodynamic measurement system. She attempted to evaluate his MPT; however, due to poor control of his laryngeal function, his values from four attempts ranged from 5 to 30 seconds. The clinician did not feel comfortable reporting an average value but recorded his range for future reference and comparison.

Perceptual Analysis

The clinician utilized the GRBAS scale for the completion of the perceptual analysis. The following are the scores in each section: G = 3, R = 3, B = 4, A = 3, S = 3. The scores on this analysis reveal that breathiness of the voice was perceived to be moderately to severely dysphonic, characterized by significant breathiness.

Chapter Summary

This chapter has provided an overview of the many types of assessments that can be completed with a child presenting with a voice disorder. The level of accessible instrumentation and technology will vary considerably by clinical location, as well. Additionally, not all of the assessment procedures described in this chapter are appropriate for every child. Clinicians should select their assessment tools and measures based on the child's age, severity of dysphonia, and voice complaints. This chapter has also provided some cautions in interpretation of measures obtained, particularly for children who have severe dysphonia yielding an aperiodic voice signal.

References

ASHA [American Speech-Language-Hearing Association]. (2004). *Preferred practice patterns for the profession of speech-language pathology.* Retrieved from http://www.asha.org/policy/PP2004-00191/#sec1.3.34.

ASHA. (2008). *Incidence and prevalence of communication disorders and hearing loss in children, 2008 edition*. Retrieved from http://www.asha.org/research/reports/children.htm.

Awan, S. N., & Roy, N. (2009). Outcomes measurement in voice disorders: Application of an acoustic index of dysphonia severity. *Journal of Speech Language and Hearing Research, 52,* 482–499.

Awan, S. N., Roy, N., & Dromey, C. (2009). Estimating dysphonia severity in continuous speech: Application of a multiple spectral/cepstral model. *Clinical Linguistics and Phonetics, 23,* 825–841.

Awan, S. N., Roy, N., Jette, M., Meltzner, G., & Hillman, R. E. (2010). Quantifying dysphonia severity using a spectral/cepstral based acoustic index: Comparisons with auditory-perceptual judgments from the CAPE-V. *Clinical Linguistics and Phonetics, 24,* 742–758.

Baker, S., Weinrich, B., Bevington, M., Schroth, K., & Schroeder, E. (2008). The effect of task type on fundamental frequency in children. *International Journal of Pediatric Otorhinolaryngology, 72,* 885–889.

Bless, D. M., Hirano, M., & Feder, R. J. (1987). Videostroboscopic evaluation of the larynx. *Ear, Nose, and Throat Journal, 66,* 289–296.

Boone, D. (1993). *The Boone voice program for children* (2nd ed.). Austin, TX: Pro-Ed.

Boseley, M. E., Cunningham, M. J., Volk, M. S., & Hartnick, C. J. (2006). Validation of the pediatric voice-related quality-of-life survey. *Archives of Otolaryngology-Head and Neck Surgery, 132,* 717–720. doi:10.1001/archotol.132.7.717

Brehm, S. B., Weinrich, B. D., Sprouse, D. C., May, S. K., & Hughes, M. R. (2012). An examination of elicitation method on fundamental frequency and repeatability of average airflow measures in children age 4:0–5:11. *Journal of Voice, 26,* 721–725.

Cheyne, H. A., Nuss, R. C., & Hillman, R. E. (1999). Electroglottography in the pediatric population. *Archives of Otolaryngology-Head & Neck Surgery, 125,* 1105–1108.

Damrose, J. F., Goldman, S. N., Groessl E. J., & Orloff, L. A. (2004). The impact of long-term botulinum toxin injections on symptom severity in patients with spasmodic dysphonia. *Journal of Voice, 18,* 415–422.

de Alarcon, A., Brehm, S. B., Kelchner, L. N., Meinzen-Derr, J., Middendorf, J., & Weinrich, B. (2009). Comparison of Pediatric Voice Handicap Index scores with perceptual voice analysis in patients following airway reconstruction. *Annals of Otology, Rhinology and Laryngology, 118,* 581–586.

Deliyski, D. D., & Hillman, R. E. (2010). State of the art laryngeal imaging: Research and clinical implications. *Current Opinions in Otolaryngology-Head and Neck Surgery, 18,* 147–152.

Deliyski, D. D., Petrushev, P. P., Bonilha, H. S., Gerlach, T. T., Martin-Harris, B., & Hillman, R. E. (2008). Clinical implication of laryngeal high speed videoendoscopy: Challenges and evolution. *Folia Phoniatrica Logopaedica, 60,* 33–44.

Finnegan, D. E. (1984). Maximum phonation time for children with normal voices. *Journal of Communication Disorders, 17,* 309–317.

Hartnick, C. J. (2002). Validation of a pediatric voice quality-of-life instrument: The Pediatric Voice Outcome Survey. *Archives of Otolaryngology-Head and Neck Surgery, 129,* 919–922.

Hartnick, C. J., Volk, M., & Cunningham, M. (2003). Establishing normative voice-related quality of life scores within the pediatric otolaryngology population. *Archives of Otolaryngology-Head and Neck Surgery, 129,* 1090–1093.

Hartnick, C. J., & Zeitels, S. M. (2005). Pediatric video laryngo-stroboscopy. *International Journal of Pediatric Otorhinolaryngology, 69,* 215–219.

Hertegård, S. (2005). What have we learned about laryngeal physiology from high-speed digital videoendoscopy? *Current Opinion in Otolaryngology-Head and Neck Surgery, 13,* 152–156.

Hirano, M. (1981). *Clinical examination of the voice.* New York, NY: Springer-Verlag.

Huber, J. E., Stathopoulos, E. T., Bormann, L. A., & Johnson, K. (1998). Effects of a circumferentially vented mask on breathing patterns of women as measured by respiratory kinematic techniques. *Journal of Speech, Language, and Hearing Research, 41*, 472–478.

Johnson, K., Brehm, S. B., Weinrich, B., Meinzen-Derr, J., & de Alarcon, A. (2011). Comparison of the Pediatric Voice Handicap Index with perceptual voice analysis in pediatric patients with vocal fold lesions. *Archives of Otolaryngology-Head and Neck Surgery, 136*, 1258–1262.

KayPENTAX Instruction Manual. (2011). Color High Speed Video System and Components, Model 9710. KayPENTAX, Montvale, NJ.

Kelchner, L. N., Brehm, S. B., Weinrich, B., Middendorf, J., de Alacron, A., Levin, L., & Elluru, R. (2010). Perceptual evaluation of severe pediatric voice disorders: Rater reliability using the consensus auditory perceptual evaluation of voice. *Journal of Voice, 24*, 441–449.

Kelchner, L. N., Weinrich, B., Brehm, S. B., Tabangin, M. E., & de Alacron, A. (2010). Characterization of supraglottic phonation in children after airway reconstruction. *Annals of Otology, Rhinology and Laryngology, 199*, 383–390.

Kempster, G. B., Gerratt, B.R., Verdolini Abbott, K., Barkmeier-Kraemer, J., & Hillman, R. E. (2009). Consensus auditory-perceptual evaluation of voice: Development of a standardized clinical protocol. *American Journal of Speech-Language Pathology, 18,* 124–132.

Laczi, E., Sussman, J. E., Stathopoulos, E. T., & Huber, J. (2005). Perceptual evaluation of hypernasality compared to HONC measures: The role of experience. *Cleft Palate-Craniofacial Journal, 42*, 202–211.

Lee, L., Stemple, J., & Glaze, L. (2005). *Quick screen for voice*. San Diego, CA: Plural Publishing.

Lee, L., Stemple, J., Glaze, L., & Kelchner, L. (2004). Quick screen for voice and supplementary documents for identifying pediatric voice disorders. *Language, Speech, and Hearing Services In Schools, 35*, 308–319.

Linders, B., Massa, G. G., Boersma, B., & Dejonckere, P. H. (1995). Fundamental voice frequency and jitter in girls and boys measured with electroglottography: Influence of age and heights. *International Journal of Pediatric Otorhinolaryngology, 33*, 61–65.

MedlinePlus/U.S. National Library of Medicine. (2013, February 20). Methlyphenidate. Retrieved from http://www.nlm.nih.gov/medline plus/druginfo/meds/a682188.html

Merati, A. L., Keppel, K., Braun, N. M., Blumin, J. H., & Kerschner, J. E. (2008). Pediatric voice-related quality of life: Findings in healthy children and in common laryngeal disorders. *Annals of Otology, Rhinology, and Laryngology, 117*, 259–262.

Meredith, M. L., Theis, S. M., McMurray, S., Zhang, Y., & Jiang, J. J. (2008). Describing pediatric dysphonia with nonlinear dynamic parameters. *International Journal of Pediatric Otorhinolaryngology, 72*, 1829–1836.

Nuss, R. C., Ward, J., Huang, L., Volk, M., & Woodnorth G. H. (2010). Correlation of vocal fold nodule size in children and perceptual assessment of voice quality. *Annals of Otology, Rhinology, and Laryngology, 119*, 651–655.

Pedersen, M. F., Moller, S., Krabbe, S., Bennett, P., & Svenstrup B. (1990). Fundamental voice frequency in female puberty measured with electroglottography during continuous speech as a secondary sex characteristic. A comparison between voice, pubertal stages, oestrogens, and androgens. *International Journal of Pediatric Otorhinolaryngology, 20*, 17–24.

Reynolds, V., Buckland, A., Bailey, J., Lipscombe, J., Nathan, E., Vijayasekaran, S., . . . French, N. (2012). Objective assessment of pediatric voice disorders with the acoustic voice quality index. *Journal of Voice, 26*, 672.e1–672.e7.

Sapienza, C. M. & Stathopoulos, E. T. (1994). Respiratory and laryngeal measures of children and women with bilateral vocal fold nodules. *Journal of Speech and Hearing Research, 37*, 1229–1243.

Schutte, H. K., Svec, J., & Sram, F. (1998). Videokymography: Research and clinical aspects. *Logopedics, Phoniatrics & Vocology, 22*, 152–156.

Shrivastav, R., & Sapienza, C. (2003). Objective measures of breathy voice quality obtained using an auditory model. *Journal of the Acoustical Society of America, 114*, 2217–2224.

Smitheran, J. R., & Hixon, T. J. (1981). A clinical method for estimating laryngeal airway resistance during vowel production. *Journal of Speech and Hearing Disorders, 46*, 138–146.

Solomon, N. P., Garlitz, S. J., & Milbrath, R. L. (2000). Respiratory and laryngeal contributions to maximum phonation duration. *Journal of Voice, 14*, 331–340.

Stathopoulos, E. T., & Sapienza, C. M. (1997). Developmental changes in laryngeal and respiratory function with variations in sound pressure level. *Journal of Speech, Language, and Hearing Research, 40*, 595–614.

Svec, J. G., & Schutte, H. K. (2012). Kymographic imaging of laryngeal vibrations. *Current Opinion in Otolaryngology-Head and Neck Surgery, 20*, 458–465.

Tavares, E. L. M., Brasolotto, A. G., Rodrigues, S. A., Benito Pessin, A. B., & Garcia Martins, R. H. (2012). Maximum phonation time and s/z ratio in a large child cohort. *Journal of Voice, 26*, 675.e1–675.e4. doi:10.1016/j.jvoice.2012.03.001

Tezcaner, C., Ozgursoy, S., Sati, I., & Dursun, G. (2009). Changes after voice therapy in objective and subjective voice measurements of pediatric patients with vocal nodules. *European Archives of Oto-Rhino-Laryngology, 266*, 1923–1927. doi:10.1007/s00405-009-1008-6

Titze, I. (1994). *Workshop on acoustic voice analysis: Summary statement.* Denver, CO: National Center for Voice and Speech.

Weinrich, B., Brehm, S. B., Knudsen, C., McBride, S., & Hughes, M. (2012). Pediatric normative data for the KayPENTAX Phonatory Aerodynamic System Model 6600. *Journal of Voice, 27*, 46–56.

Weinrich, B., Salz, B., & Hughes, M. (2005). Aerodynamic measurements: Normative data for children ages 6:0-10:11 Years. *Journal of Voice, 19*, 326–339.

Wolfe, V., Fitch, J., & Martin, D. (1997). Acoustic measures of dysphonic severity across and within voice types. *Folia Phoniatrica et Logopaedica, 49*, 292–299.

Zraick, R., Skaggs, S., & Montague, J. (2000). The effect of task on determination of habitual pitch. *Journal of Voice, 14*, 484–489.

Zur, K. B., Cotton, S., Kelchner, L., Baker, S., Weinrich, B., and Lee, L. (2007). Pediatric Voice Handicap Index Index (pVHI): A new tool for evaluating pediatric dysphonia. *International Journal of Pediatric Otorhinolaryngology, 71*, 77–82.

APPENDIX 5–A

Initial Intake History Form

Medical Record Number _____   Today's Date ___/___/_____
Patient Birth Date _____/_____/_____

Why was your child referred to the Voice Clinic? Please check all that apply:

☐   My child is hoarse.

☐   My child has a quiet voice.

☐   My child's physician referred us to this clinic.

☐   Other: _____

☐

Who referred your child? _____

MEDICAL HISTORY

Was your child full-term?   *Yes   No*   If no, how many weeks gestation? _____ weeks.
Does your child have any of the following medical conditions?

	Yes	*No*	*Unknown*
Down Syndrome	☐	☐	☐
Eosinophilic Esophagitis (EE)	☐	☐	☐
Head Trauma	☐	☐	☐
Intellectual Disability	☐	☐	☐
Cerebral Palsy	☐	☐	☐

	Currently			In the past		
	Yes	*No*	*Unknown*	*Yes*	*No*	*Unknown*
Gastrointestinal Reflux	☐	☐	☐	☐	☐	☐
Cancer	☐	☐	☐	☐	☐	☐
Asthma	☐	☐	☐	☐	☐	☐
Swallowing Disorder	☐	☐	☐	☐	☐	☐
Heart Condition	☐	☐	☐	☐	☐	☐
BPD	☐	☐	☐	☐	☐	☐
Other Pulmonary Disease	☐	☐	☐	☐	☐	☐
Other (Please describe)	☐	☐	☐	☐	☐	☐

My child is exposed to cigarette smoke: *Daily   Occasionally   Never*

How much of the following beverages does your child drink per day? (1 cup is approx. 8 oz.)
- ☐ Water _____ cups
- ☐ Juice _____cups
- ☐ Milk _____cups
- ☐ Soda/Pop _____cups

Airway History

Was your child ever intubated (breathing tube through mouth)?   *Yes   No   Unknown*
   If yes, how long? _____days_____weeks_____months

Did your child require multiple intubations?   *Yes   No   Unknown*

Did you child require a tracheostomy tube?   *Yes   No   Unknown*
   If yes, how long? _____days_____weeks_____months

Does your child currently have a tracheostomy tube?   *Yes   No*
   If yes, does your child use a Passy-Muir valve?   *Yes   No*
   If yes, how many hours is the valve worn during the day?_____

Does your child have any of the following symptoms?

	Always	*Sometimes*	*Never*
Stridor (noise when breathing)	☐	☐	☐
Shortness of breath during exercise	☐	☐	☐
Shortness of breath during speech	☐	☐	☐
Snoring	☐	☐	☐

VOICE HISTORY

Does your child have the following symptoms related to his or her voice?

	Always	*Sometimes*	*Never*
Frequent hoarseness.	☐	☐	☐
The volume of the voice is too soft.	☐	☐	☐
The volume of the voice is too loud.	☐	☐	☐
The voice sounds breathy or airy.	☐	☐	☐
The pitch of the voice is too high.	☐	☐	☐
The pitch of the voice is too low.	☐	☐	☐
Pain associated with voice use.	☐	☐	☐
Increased effort to use the voice.	☐	☐	☐
Fatigue during/after voice use.	☐	☐	☐

Does your child's voice vary in quality throughout the day (e.g., worse in the morning or worse in the evening)?   *Yes   No*   If yes, please describe:_____
_____

Do you, your family, or others have a hard time understanding what you child says?   *Yes   No*
If yes, please describe: _____
_____

Describe your child's typical amount of talking during the day: *Excessive   Normal   Minimal*

Does your child overuse his/her voice during the day (screaming, shouting, crying, cheering)? *Yes   No*   If yes, please describe: _____

Is your child a singer?   *Yes   No*

If yes, does your child take singing lessons?   *Yes   No*

SWALLOWING

Has your child ever had difficulty with feeding and/or swallowing?   *Yes   No   Unknown*

If yes, has your child ever:

	Yes	*No*	*Unknown*
Been NPO (not allowed to eat/drink by mouth)?	☐	☐	☐
Required a G Tube for nutrition?	☐	☐	☐
Had a restricted diet for the type of liquid or food consumed?	☐	☐	☐
Coughed/choked during or after drinking/eating?	☐	☐	☐
Had a voice change after drinking/eating?	☐	☐	☐
Refused to drink or eat by mouth?	☐	☐	☐
Had multiple lung infections due to swallowing difficulty?	☐	☐	☐

DEVELOPMENTAL HISTORY

Were developmental milestones for: Motor skills (walking)   *Normal   Delayed*

Communication (talking)   *Normal   Delayed*

What is your child's current grade in school? _____

Is your child making appropriate progress in school (academically and socially)? *Yes   No   Unknown*

Has your child ever received speech therapy?   *Yes   No   Unknown*

Is your child currently receiving speech therapy?   *Yes   No   Unknown*

If yes, what has been or is the focus of this therapy? Please check all that apply:

In the past

☐ Swallowing
☐ Articulation development
☐ Language development
☐ Voice quality

Currently

☐ Swallowing
☐ Articulation development
☐ Language development
☐ Voice quality

Other information that you feel is useful for the voice team:

Note: Modified and used courtesy of Cincinnati Children's Hospital Medical Center, Division of Speech-Language Pathology.

APPENDIX 5–B

DVD Table of Contents

Perceptual analysis practice with CAPE-V sentences
Laryngeal imaging evaluation practice with stroboscopy ratings
Example of completing acoustic measurement protocol
Example of completing CAPE-V sentences
Example of completing aerodynamic measurement protocol
Explanation of child preparation for rigid endoscopy.

CHAPTER 6

A Collaborative Approach to Treatment

Overview

This chapter describes treatment using a collaborative model and addresses the specific needs of solo and school-based practitioners. Both traditional behavioral techniques and new models of delivery, including telehealth and gaming, are discussed. The adult voice research literature provides several clinical studies for direct therapy techniques (e.g., Vocal Function Exercises, Resonant Voice Therapy) that are included in this chapter (Roy et al., 2001, 2003; Sabol, Lee, & Stemple, 1995; Stemple, Lee, D'Amico, & Pickup, 1994). In contrast, the pediatric voice literature is lacking in evidence-based research for specific treatment techniques. Moreover, large-scale clinical trials have not been conducted. Clinicians with minimal expertise in pediatric voice care should look for evidence of support for particular techniques based on provision of competent clinical care by experienced speech-language pathologists (SLPs).

Collaborative Treatment Model

A collaborative treatment approach indicates that individuals with different backgrounds and areas of expertise come together to assess the patient and develop a management strategy. Depending on the issues involved, voice-care teams may include SLPs, general practitioners, surgeons, medical or radiation oncologists, nurses, social workers, occupational therapists, dieticians, and pharmacists. These members, with varied but complementary experience, qualifications, and skills, offer specific contributions to the delivery of quality care received by the patient. Optimally, the team is interdisciplinary, comprising professionals from different disciplines who meet and discuss patient care to develop a unified management plan. Alternatively, the team may be multidisciplinary, consisting of individuals working independently with no regular team meetings. This may produce fragmented patient care, with conflicting information provided to the patients and families.

There are multiple providers involved in the treatment process for children with voice and/or airway disorders, which warrants a collaborative treatment model for best practice care. The SLP is a primary treatment provider for pediatric cases and often serves as team manager. Within the core of the team, the SLP partners with a pediatric otolaryngologist and nurse for voice disorders or with a pulmonologist/allergist, pediatric otolaryngologist, and nurse for upper airway disorders.

Individuals with reflux disorders may require the care of a gastroenterologist.

Solo or School-Based Practitioner

The SLP can provide treatment services in a variety of settings, including hospitals, private clinics, private practice, home health care, and schools. Typically, in medical settings, the proximity of care providers can enhance the collaborative process. Often, the solo or school-based practitioner can be challenged by the lack of communication between caregivers in various disciplines. This may stymie a collaborative treatment model. When this occurs, it becomes the SLP's responsibility to communicate with the other professionals who have participated in the child's care.

Making the Case

Treatment for childhood voice disorders within the educational setting may not be provided. School districts throughout the United States vary in their decision-making process regarding enrollment in therapy following a medical referral for a child with a voice disorder. Questions arise regarding whether the school district has a financial obligation to pay for the evaluation when it is recommended by the school SLP. Enrollment priority is often given to children with communication disorders that are educationally handicapping as opposed to children with communication disorders that stem from medical issues but are not educationally handicapping. Ruddy and Sapienza (2004) reported that perceptions among clinicians regarding eligibility decisions for voice treatment in the schools under the Individuals with Disabilities Education Act (IDEA) amendments of 1997 (P.L. 105-17) are open for interpretation. This results in children with voice disorders having inconsistent access to treatment. Within the educational setting, if a child presents with only a voice disorder, professionals involved may not view it as an educational handicap significant enough to warrant individual treatment. Each individual case may need the support of the SLP to justify the potential negative effects of a voice disorder on a child's academic participation. For example, severe roughness, breathiness, or low volume may interfere with overall intelligibility and significantly restrict a child's participation in the classroom. If other speech and/or language disorders are present, voice is often not the primary focus of the communication intervention. Consequently, voice disorders in children may go untreated in an educational setting (Weinrich, 2002).

Considering the relative lack of services for pediatric voice disorders provided in the schools, Kahane and Mayo (1989) called for mass screenings of school-aged children and implementation of programs to teach about and prevent vocally abusive behaviors. However, the call for prevention was unanswered, with data from 1994 indicating that only 1% of school SLPs reported conducting a prevention program within a 2-year period (McNamara & Perry, 1994). An alternative to implementation of a prevention program in the schools is to encourage members of the community, such as physicians and local media, to provide families with information regarding vocal health (Weinrich, 2002). Prevention of pediatric voice disorders can be accomplished by educating children and their caregivers about vocally abusive behaviors, which is clearly preferable to providing treatment after a disorder has developed.

Both prevention and treatment for voice disorders are needed in the school setting. As SLPs increase their awareness of and knowledge about pediatric voice disorders and the unique treatment characteristics, they will be better equipped to advocate for appropriate prevention and treatment programs. The ultimate goal of this effort is the healthy vocal development of the children they serve (Weinrich, 2002).

Communicating with Teachers and Others

Interactions between the SLP and teacher regarding risks and needs of students with voice disorders are important. Given the amount of time children spend at school, teachers have a significant role in shaping students' future directions. Students' academic achievements, quality of life, self-perceptions, social interactions, and future occupations may be directly affected by teachers' attitudes toward them (Becker & Maiman, 1985; Overby, Carrell, & Bernthal, 2007).

Teachers' perceptions of their students lead to certain expectations that may have positive or negative influences on the student (Babad, 1993; Good, 1987; Ripich, 1989). Therefore, it is possible that within a classroom situation the presence of a voice disorder alone may make a student more vulnerable to academic and social biases (Becker & Maiman, 1985; Overby et al., 2007). Zacharias, Kelchner, and Creaghead (2013) report that teachers' overall attitudes and ratings of several social/emotional and health related personality traits (emotional adjustment, happiness, health, likability, sociability, employableness, strength of character) were more negative in adolescent females with a mild, moderate, or severe voice disorder compared with adolescent females with no voice disorder. These researchers concluded that a voice disorder may negatively impact expectations of teachers, placing the student at risk for negative educational, social, and occupational outcomes.

Informing teachers, SLPs, students, and families about these potential subtle biases

that teachers may have toward those with a voice disorder is important for each student's overall well-being. This knowledge may provide support for services and assist students with voice disorders to advocate for themselves.

Pediatric Voice Disorders and Their Identification Under IDEA

Ruddy and Sapienza (2004) described changes occurring in the population with whom school-based SLPs work. Advances in medical technology and life-sustaining procedures, along with the current focus on placing children with disabilities in the least restrictive educational environment, have altered school-based SLPs' caseloads to include children with congenital, surgical, or medically fragile conditions. Clinicians often have questions about how to best help these students function in the classroom. They also question whether treatment for voice disorders falls under the provisions of IDEA. Indeed, Part B of IDEA states that eligibility for services is determined based on whether or not the disability has a negative impact on the child's academic performance.

Policy statements from the Department of Education and the Office of Special Education Programs (OSEP) have provided clarification that voice disorders can have a negative impact on academic performance. Voice and laryngeal disorders in school-aged children can limit their participation in classroom activities that require speaking, negatively impact peer interactions, and restrict their participation in athletic activities and/or vigorous play. Finally, adolescents participating in vocational or co-op programs in high school may feel inhibited by their voice disorder and make long-term career decisions based on early negative experiences in the workplace (Ruddy & Sapienza, 2004). It is clear that vocal health has an impact on a child's academic experience. Therefore, it is the role of the SLP to advocate for a thorough evaluation of these children and to provide appropriate treatment as needed.

Access to Professional Care

Following diagnosis of a voice disorder, a referral from a physician for voice therapy is necessary prior to enrollment in a treatment program. This referral may be made by the primary medical care provider, i.e., pediatrician or general practice physician, or preferably by an otolaryngologist. The SLP has a professional responsibility to meet basic competencies in the treatment of voice disorders when enrolling a child in therapy.

One example of establishing competencies in a larger medical setting is seen in the Voice Specialty Team, Division of Speech-Language Pathology at Cincinnati Children's Hospital Medical Center, Cincinnati, Ohio, which has developed templates that include competency modules for Level I and Level II SLPs. The Level I SLP must demonstrate the specified clinical knowledge and skill competencies to provide treatment, counsel, and referrals as determined by a mentor SLP, who has qualified for Level II. The Level II SLP has met all the knowledge and skills competencies to provide treatment, counsel, and referral independently. The voice competencies include knowledge of: laryngeal anatomy/physiology; laryngeal anomalies; etiologies of voice disorders; effects of voice disorders on communication, behavior, and social interactions; medical and nutritional factors related to voice disorders; perceptual and instrumental voice assessment process; components of a successful voice interview/evaluation; a variety of therapy approaches for voice disorders; and counseling skills to provide patient/family support.

Establishing a Connection With Child and Family

One universal role of SLPs is to gain the confidence of the child and family regarding their knowledge and expertise in treating the voice disorder. In order to establish a connection with the child, it is important to know the value that the child and family place upon the child's voice disorder as it relates to daily routines.

In addition to the SLP connecting with the child, the role of the family in the child's progress during therapy has been documented in the literature. Nienkerke-Springer, McAllister, and Sundberg (2005) implemented a holistic therapy program, the SYGESTI (Systemisch gestorte Stimme; System-Related Voice Disorders), based on the idea that some pediatric voice disorders stem from developmental problems and/or social context and life situations. The program included minimal direct voice therapy, focusing instead on discussing current family interactions and setting goals for improved communication among members of the child's social context. The results of the study showed that this 14-week program, which heavily incorporated the family in the child's treatment, did increase the vocal quality of the children.

Indirect Treatment Methods

Indirect treatment techniques seek to eliminate vocal trauma by modifying behaviors beyond voicing. Clinicians treating pediatric voice disorders often counsel children and their parents about ways to avoid vocally abusive behaviors. For example, children with voice disorders should have preferential seating in the classroom in order to reduce demands placed on their voice when interacting with the teacher during class time. Also, close proximity to the teacher may help to decrease the amount of extra speaking and whispering with classmates throughout the school day. Teaching turn-taking behaviors during conversation can help to eliminate attempts to talk over someone else, an act generally requiring loud, forceful phonation. Children can also be encouraged to use a soft voice for play and be taught how to shout in a manner less abusive to their vocal folds. Finally, a family in the habit of shouting to one another within the home should consider instituting new habits of walking to within proximity of the listener before speaking. This practice would encourage the child with a voice disorder to speak only within close listening range with his or her family members and could also generalize to his or her interactions with others.

Children with voice disorders also benefit from hygienic voice therapy. Counseling for vocal hygiene involves talking with the child and parents to identify phonotraumatic behaviors. Vocally abusive behaviors more often seen in children include screaming and vocal play noises, such as loud dinosaur growls and truck sounds. Similar to adults, children might engage in frequent throat clearing and vocally abusive coughing or persistent talking in a loud voice. Hydration is an important element for a healthy vocal mechanism, and hydration counseling is typically part of vocal hygiene counseling (Stemple, Glaze, & Klaben, 2010). Hydration in children may raise particular challenges, as children might "forget" to ask for a drink when engrossed in play. Also, children spend as much of their day in school as adults spend at work. Therefore, the clinician should ask about the child's access to water and the restroom during the school day. A conversation between the clinician and the child's teacher about the child's increased hydration needs can help the child to feel more comfortable about asking for more water or a restroom break during class.

See Appendix 6–A for a sample handout regarding general guidelines for vocal hygiene.

Once phonotraumatic behaviors have been identified, the clinician should explain how the behaviors are impacting vocal anatomy and physiology. The clinician, child, and parents could then devise a means to track these behaviors between therapy sessions and discuss ways to change or eliminate the behavior. See Appendix 6–B for a sample vocal hygiene record form.

The presence of gastroesophageal reflux (GER) or laryngopharyngeal reflux (LPR), diagnosed by a physician, can be contributing factors for a voice disorder. GER or LPR occur when contents from the stomach, or stomach acid, reflux into the posterior portion of the larynx. This acid is irritating to the laryngeal tissues, and frequent exposure to the refluxed fluids can cause edema, feeling of a lump in the throat, hoarseness, and vocally abusive behaviors, such as chronic coughing and throat clearing. The physician will determine whether medication should be prescribed. The pediatric voice clinician should counsel children and their parents about controlling reflux by remaining upright for at least half an hour after eating; eating frequent, small meals throughout the day; avoiding caffeine and other foods that contribute to reflux, such as tomato-based products; raising the head of the bed (from the floor level); and eliminating pre-bedtime snacks. See Appendix 6–C for a sample handout with more information about gastroesophageal reflux, its causes, and impact on the voice.

Direct Treatment Methods

There are numerous direct treatment methods that are employed to facilitate normal voice characteristics in children with voice disorders. The techniques that follow share some commonalities, although each technique is unique in its design specificity. All techniques are meant to be tailored to the individual needs of each child with a voice disorder. For sample demonstrations of the majority of treatment methods described below, see the accompanying DVD.

Vocal Function Exercises

Stemple and colleagues (2010) describe Vocal Function Exercises (VFEs) as a treatment technique used to improve the balance between respiration, phonation, and resonance. These voice therapy exercises mimic elements of physical therapy in that the clinician seeks to rehabilitate the larynx, comprising cartilages, joints, muscles, and connective tissue, to a balanced and efficient system for movement. The exercises promote rehabilitation of the larynx by strengthening and coordinating the laryngeal muscles. The increased efficiency of this system allows for improved phonation.

Before beginning the exercises, the clinician should counsel the child about behaviors that will enhance the benefits of VFEs. While performing the exercises, the child should adopt a posture that facilitates supportive abdominal breathing. The tone placement should have a forward focus, and tone onset should be easy, instead of containing hard glottal attacks. Counseling for healthy voicing is an ongoing process, as the child needs time to develop these facilitative habits. Therefore, each session should begin with an assessment and a purposeful discussion about the child's ability to achieve the correct manner of production. All exercises should be performed as quietly as possible and repeated twice. At the onset of treatment, VFEs should be performed twice daily (A.M. and P.M.), but this dosage is reduced as the child progresses through the program. At home, practice should be indi-

cated on a record form, which the child brings to therapy and discusses with the clinician (Stemple et al., 2010). See Appendices 6–D and 6–E for a sample Vocal Function Exercises Home Instructions handout and a sample data form.

Vocal Function Exercises (VFE)—Four Steps

After correct posture and breathing patterns are established, the four steps of the Vocal Function Exercises, as described by Stemple et al. (2010), are implemented. Each step is performed twice during a treatment session. Adaptations that can be made for children are provided in the next section of this chapter.

Step 1. Therapy begins with a *warm-up* exercise that is timed. The goal of the warm-up exercise is to increase the duration of a sustained tone. The child produces the vowel /i/ with a nasal tone for as long as possible. (Instruct the child to take a deep breath through the nose and make a soft production.) The younger children and female adolescents typically produce a tone at the musical note F above middle C, while the adolescent males may produce F below middle C. This note can vary depending upon the comfortable range of the child. It should be a note that is in the higher end of the child's comfortable range. Compare the duration in seconds of the child's longest sustained tone during the warm-up exercise with the child's ideal value. The ideal value can be calculated by dividing the child's expiratory airflow volume by 80 (airflow rate; mL/s). This value (80 mL/s) represents the most efficient use of the vocal system by the child. (For example, if the expiratory lung volume was 1600 milliliters divided by 80, the ideal time would be 20 seconds.) If the expiratory lung volume is not known, ask the child to take a deep breath through the nose and make a soft "skinny S" sound for as long as possible, timing this event. That time would represent the target value for the sustained tone. (As the child completes the VFE therapy, his or her duration for sustaining the warm-up note should move closer to the ideal time.) Throughout this exercise, the clinician will monitor the child's posture, breathing, tone onset, and tone focus.

Step 2. The next exercise aims to *stretch* the vocal folds and provide greater control of the cricothyroid muscles. First, the child glides from a low note to his or her highest on the word "whoop" or "knoll." Lip buzzes or tongue trills are also acceptable and initially may be easier for the child. The child should strive to glide from low to high pitch with no breaks in voicing.

Step 3. The next exercise is a *contracting* movement that focuses on the thyroarytenoid musculature. Here, the child glides from a high note to his or her lowest note, again using "whoop," "knoll," "boom," lip buzzes, or tongue trills. As with the stretching exercise, the goal is to perform the maneuver without a disruption in voicing. The child should be cautioned not to drop into the glottal fry register while gliding down to the lowest note.

Step 4. Finally, *power exercises* work to strengthen the laryngeal adductory muscles. The child produces five notes within his or her comfortable range (ideally C-D-E-F-G), sustaining each tone for as long as possible and performing each note two times. As softly as possible, but not breathily, the child produces the word "old" without the "d" while sustaining each note. The tone should be forward focused and without tension. The five notes can be modified—B-C-D-E-F or A-B-C-D-E, etc.—depending on the individual's comfortable range.

Facilitating VFEs for Home Instruction

When requesting that Vocal Function Exercises be performed at home, it is very important to provide the family with clear instructions (Appendix 6–D), as many visuals

as possible, and reminders to record all times collected during exercises on an easy-to-follow chart or record form (Appendix 6–E). Providing a record form that is returned each session will enhance better compliance with clinical recommendations. Parents should encourage their child to drink water, sit up straight or stand, and take their time when completing the exercises at home.

In order for the child and parents to understand the VFE procedure, the clinician should describe all steps in a *language-friendly* manner, as stated below. Additionally, provide parents with a CD that has a clinician modeling the exercises with notes that are appropriate for their child.

- (Step 1) Indicate that the first exercise requires their child to match a note and produce the letter "E" for as long as possible, remembering to record the child's time.
- (Steps 2 and 3) Describe the procedure for "stretching the voice up and back down." While "stretching up" from a low note to their highest note on the word "whoop," children may begin with their hands together and slowly pull them apart until their arms are fully outstretched when they reach their highest note. The opposite procedure may be followed when "stretching down" from a high note to their lowest pitch on the word "boom." (As stated previously, modifications of the *stretches/contractions* include the use of lip buzzes and tongue trills.) Another technique to make the exercises more fun and motivating is to instruct the children to stretch their voice up or down while pretending to be a siren, an owl, a train, a kite, a parachute, or an apple falling from a tree.
- (Step 4) Tell children to make their lips "buzz like a bee" or "sound like an owl," when they produce a note for as long as possible while using the word "ol." As this is a timed exercise, some children are

motivated to "break their record." Some children have difficulty matching pitches while performing these *power exercises.* If this is the case, the exercises should be amended to include low-, medium-, and high-pitched notes. The relative relationship may be easier for some children to understand, and they will still be performing the exercises throughout their vocal range.

Resonance Therapy

Resonance Therapy is a modified form of Resonant Voice Therapy (RVT), which is a holistic therapy approach that seeks to directly modify the tone focus of the patient to a forward focus production. In general, resonant voice may be described as the combination of simultaneous oral vibratory sensations and easy phonation (Stemple et al., 2010). The therapy technique facilitates forward focus by progressing through a series of exercises requiring nasal to nasal/oral productions. By practicing nasalized speech, the patient become familiar with "buzzy sensations" in the facial region. These sensations help the patients to attend to the location of their tone focus during speech tasks and develop the skills necessary to manipulate the placement of their speaking tone. The patient's goal in therapy is to maintain a clear, strong voice with a small amount of effort in order to diminish the risk of vocal fold injury (Stemple et al., 2010). Berry and colleagues (2001) argued that the glottal posture assumed during RVT maximizes the efficiency of energy for voicing. The RVT technique is based on the work of a performing arts trainer, Lessac (1997), who argued that the placement of the voice contributes to or hinders the balance of the laryngeal mechanism with respiration and resonance. Additional contributors to RVT include Katherine Verdolini Abbott, with the current Lessac-Madsen Resonant Voice Training (Verdolini Abbott, 1998).

Although the focus of RVT is resonance, modification of resonance characteristics will have a positive impact on respiration and phonation. When performing RVT, the patient aims to maintain easy voicing, beginning with basic speech sounds and progressing to phonation for conversation. During therapy tasks, the patient should perceive vibratory sensations in the area of the anterior alveolar ridge to the nares and nasal cavity. As RVT training is experiential and based upon the processing of sensory information, patients will continuously be asked to monitor the "feeling" they are sensing and to concentrate on the auditory feedback they are receiving. The treatment approach stresses the importance of training through repetition, but also emphasizes that repetition tasks must be performed with precision in order to gain the benefits possible from the exercises (Stemple et al., 2010).

Resonance Therapy—Eight Steps

The eight steps of Resonance Therapy presented below are child-based adaptations of RVT described by Stemple and colleagues (2010). Before beginning Resonance Therapy, children should warm up their neck, shoulder, jaw, floor of mouth, lips, tongue, and pharyngeal muscles by stretching, yawning, and massaging these areas. Supportive abdominal breathing should be established.

1. Step 1. This step begins with a sigh exercise. The child should say "holm-molm-molm-molm . . .", as if sighing. The sigh should be produced with extreme forward focus and end in a relaxed posture.
2. Step 2. The child should produce "molm-molm-molm" as a chant using a comfortable note, first varying only the rate of production (slow-fast-slow), then only the intensity of production (soft-loud-soft).
3. Step 3. This step uses speech-like intona-

tion, by varying the rate, pitch, and loudness of "molm." The varied repetition of "molm" should mimic a sentence, as if you are speaking to someone.

4. Step 4. The next step is to chant nasal phoneme-loaded sentences on a comfortable note (e.g., Mary made me mad). The sentence length can be modified to a phrase for the child, but still should contain nasal phonemes (e.g., *my mom* or *my money*). This is followed by chanting these same sentences, but with exaggerated speech-like intonation. Care should be taken that the child does not drop into the glottal fry register at the end of the sentence tasks. Lastly, each sentence is produced in a natural, speech-like manner.

5. Step 5. This step consists of contrasting voiced and voiceless phonemes, as well as nasal and oral consonants. The child chants "mamapapa" using a comfortable note, first varying the rate (slow-fast-slow), then varying the intensity of productions (soft-loud-soft). This is followed by speech-like intonation, with variations of rate, pitch, and loudness of "mamapapa." The varied repetition of "mamapapa" should mimic a sentence, as if you were speaking to someone.

6. Step 6. Sentences that emphasize the voiced and voiceless phoneme contrast—for example, "Mom may put Paul on the moon"—are chanted on a comfortable note. Again, the sentence length can be modified for the child. This is followed by chanting these same sentences, but with exaggerated speech-like intonation. Again, care should be taken that the child does not drop into the glottal fry register at the end of the sentence tasks. Lastly, each sentence is produced in a natural, speech-like manner.

7. Step 7. The child and/or clinician selects a target sentence from a list of sentences with five to seven syllables. The child pro-

duces the selected sentence with a forward focus tone and natural inflection. If the forward focus tone cannot be maintained, use chanting and extra inflection.

8. Step 8. This step includes reading and conversation tasks. The clinician provides sentences with varied lengths and paragraph length readings, which are appropriate for the child's reading ability. The child reads a passage that has been marked with phrase markers for breathing. While reading the paragraph the first time, she or he should exaggerate a forward focus tone and clearly separate phrases with nasal inhalation. The child should read the paragraph a second time, with a more natural tone and without the phrase marker cues for inhalation.

Step 8 advances the child into generalization of forward focus tone with conversational speech. Therapy activities should elicit conversational speech and allow the clinician to monitor speech production for phonotraumatic behaviors, such as hard glottal attack or glottal fry register. The child progresses from using forward focus tone in conversation within the context of therapy to real-world contexts. A conversational environment outside of therapy may include loud background noise and other distractions. Approaching this nontherapy environment with the clinician allows the child to learn compensatory strategies before facing these challenges alone. Step 8 is a time for the clinician to challenge the child and prepare him or her for healthy vocal function in the future.

In order to accomplish generalization of a healthy voice, the child should practice the exercises at home in increments of 8 to 10 minutes several times per day. This length of daily practice is considered minimum and can be increased. Recording performance of the home exercises encourages compliance. As in therapy, the child should begin with stretches to warm up, as well as the basic chanting-sigh exercise, prior to performing the exercise step(s) appropriate to his or her level in therapy. See Appendix 6–F for a sample handout with instructions for practicing Resonance Therapy exercises at home. Appendix 6–G provides a sample data form for use with home practice.

Methods Based on Semiocclusion of the Vocal Tract

Methods that utilize semiocclusion of the vocal tract to increase vocal efficiency are useful in pediatric voice therapy. Semiocclusion of the vocal tract and its impact on the disordered voice is reviewed by Titze (2006). Efficient voicing lessens the vibratory impact of the vocal folds and therefore decreases mechanical trauma to their upper tissue layers. By decreasing this vocal stress, vocal fold edema and possibly lesions, such as nodules, are given the opportunity to heal.

Flow Phonation

Flow phonation therapy is the outgrowth of theories related to semiocclusion (Gauffin & Sundberg, 1989; Stone & Casteel, 1982). The following three exercises constitute activities of flow phonation therapy. The activities provide the child some biofeedback regarding vocal productions (Gartner-Schmidt, 2010).

Begin with a *gargling* activity. (For young children, this activity works better in the bathtub or outside in a wading pool.) The child sips a small amount of water, tilts chin upward, and gargles the water without voicing, producing many water bubbles. This procedure can be repeated multiple times, pausing between exercises. This is followed by the child performing the same activity, but with voicing (making a gargling sound). Instruc-

tions are given to relax the throat and attempt to make bubbles pop out of the mouth. Next, the child gargles while pitch gliding up and down her vocal range. Again, the participant should be relaxed. Finally, the child begins to gargle, then rolls her head forward while continuing to gargle and closing the mouth. Once the mouth has closed, the gargle sounds will resonate through the nasal cavity and sound like a hum. At this time, the child swallows the water, breathes, and begins to voice "m-m-m-m." This is followed by imitation of the clinician's model for /m/ + vowel syllables. Voicing words with any nasal phoneme in the initial position leads to continued speech tasks with efficient voicing (Gartner-Schmidt, 2010; Stone & Casteel, 1982).

The second activity in this series is *cup bubble blowing*. The child is given a clear plastic cup approximately two-thirds filled with water. She places her mouth on the cup as if to drink, but tips it back only until the water touches her top lip. After drawing a nasal breath, she first blows bubbles into the cup without voicing, then with voicing. It is important that when the child switches to the voiced bubble blowing, she maintains the same bubble activity as seen without voicing. Next, she blows bubbles into the cup while gliding up and down in pitch. The fourth step involves the child blowing bubbles again with voice, but this time slowly removing the cup of water and continuing the vocalization to produce an "oh-h-h" or "oo-oo-oo" sound with a relaxed and breathy quality. The child takes a breath. Then she repeats the same "oh-h-h" or "oo-oo-oo" sound (Gartner-Schmidt, 2010; Stone & Casteel, 1982).

The /u/ *prolongation* exercise uses the movement of tissue paper as a means for providing biofeedback. A strip of tissue paper is grasped near the top between the index and middle finger. The child holds the paper in front of her face and blows into the tissue with puckered lips (voiceless /u/), causing the tissue to become parallel with the floor. The activity is repeated several times. After these repetitions, the child blows on the tissue again, but once it becomes parallel with the floor, she adds voicing while keeping the tissue parallel with the floor. After several repetitions at this level, the voicing and blowing begin simultaneously and once the tissue is parallel, the child says "one." If the voiced word is relaxed and effortless, continue counting. Continue the same procedure of blowing and voicing, followed by "wh" and "h" questions, instead of numbers. Follow voiceless phrases with voiced phrases, using the same technique (Gartner-Schmidt, 2010; Stone & Casteel, 1982). The /u/ prolongation can be included with the cup bubble blowing/straw phonation exercise for young children.

It is important to start this series of exercises with the activity that is easiest for the child, which is most likely the *gargling* or *cup bubble blowing*. However, the clinician can vary the series of activities depending on the child's performance. It is recommended that the child practice the exercises several times per day for 8 to 10 minutes, and a parent should log the exercise attempts (Gartner-Schmidt, 2010; Stone & Casteel, 1982).

Additional Semiocclusion Techniques

Straw phonation is another technique based on the theory of semiocclusion (Titze, 2006). Here, straws of varying diameter are placed between the lips and used for phonation. The vocal folds are slightly separated with high lung pressure as one blows air into the straw. This is easier to perform with a larger straw, such as a drinking straw rather than a stirring straw. All the steps in this technique use /ol/ as the vocal production. The child begins by producing /ol/ with voicing through the straw. This is followed by pitch glides from low to high and vice versa. Then, the glides are produced with an accented voice produced by rapid up and down voicing as she continues up the scale. Last, the child produces the musical notes from her favorite song. Ingo Titze has produced online videos (Vocal Straw Exercise, YouTube; http://www.youtube.com/watch?v=0xYDvwvmBIM), in which he demonstrates this technique, which has roots in northern Europe dating back several hundred years. Titze (2006) has argued that straw phonation is the method most likely to have high compliance because exercises can easily be done in many contexts due to the portability of the straw and the minimal sound that straw phonation makes, which draws less attention to the practice. Additionally, the resulting sound is nonspeech, which also draws little attention to the person performing the exercise. Finally, the method is efficient, as the desired effects of the semioccluded vocal tract can be achieved in the least amount of time.

Heavy use of nasal consonants is also a form of therapy based on the concept of semiocclusion. With the mouth closed and the velar port open, the nasal cavity takes on the role of the vocal tract with the nostrils providing the semiocclusion. Both VFEs and Resonant Voice Therapy are concrete manifestations of the theory of semiocclusion in practice (Titze, 2006). These techniques use abdominal support and reduce a pressed voice by diminishing laryngeal (throat) effort and increasing a lighter, buzzing tone for the voice.

Also operating within the notion of the semioccluded vocal tract is the LaxVox therapy designed by Denizoglu and Sihvo (2010). These authors recommend this therapy method for patients with muscle tension dysphonia, functional dysphonia, vocal fold paralysis, and vocal fold lesions (polyps and nodules). This is another procedure that entails using a straw or flexible tube with a glass of water. The clinician helps to position the child's head, neck, and torso in a manner that encourages relaxation and that is ideal for phonation. The child then elongates her lips and seals them onto the rim of the glass around the straw in a /u/ posture. Without voicing, the child exhales into the glass. The procedure is then repeated, but with voicing of /u/. In the next step, the procedure continues without water. Finally, the straw is eliminated and the child transitions to employing this phonatory posture to the production of words, phrases, and conversation. According to Denizoglu and Sihvo, this technique is thought to improve laryngeal glottic closure.

Another therapy technique using semiocclusion of the vocal tract is *lip buzzes*. Lip buzzes are used as a vocal warm-up exercise to increase breath support and elongate the vocal folds, as well as the amplitude of their mucosal wave, without an increase in phonotrauma. The child begins by producing a sustained, voiced lip buzz at a comfortable note. The child then repeats the sustained tone, but at three progressively higher pitches. Then, the child slowly glides from a low to a high pitch several times, each time attempting to extend her pitch range. Finally, the child returns to the comfortable note used for the first exercise and in one breath begins the lip buzz softly, builds to a moderately loud sound, then fades to a soft volume. This process of careful crescendo and diminuendo is called a *messa di voce* maneuver. The child should maintain control throughout the exercise and not fade quickly in the transition from a moderately loud to a soft buzz. The child repeats this step several times, each at a progressively higher pitch. Some children may have difficulty achieving and maintaining the lip buzz throughout the exercises. If this is the case, encourage them to relax the lips and focus on maintaining even breath support originating from the abdominal mus-

cles (Behrman, 2008). Application of lip buzz techniques for pediatric voice therapy can improve participation for some children who find them engaging.

Additional Treatment Techniques

The Casper-Stone Confidential Flow Therapy (CSCFT) promoted by Katherine Verdolini Abbott emphasizes slightly greater vocal abductions during phonation without semiocclusion. She teaches this approach as part of the Voice Therapy Spectrum workshop that she developed and conducts. This workshop emphasizes the application of treatment approaches based on the individual needs and characteristics of the patient. CSCFT is contrasted with the Lessac-Madsen Resonant Voice Therapy (LMRVT), which emphasizes full vocal fold closure, as well as semiocclusion of the vocal tract. Although both methods incorporate motor learning principles and stress the importance of patient compliance, the clinician and patient make decisions about implementation of one approach versus the other based on specific pathology and patient preference (Verdolini Abbott, 2012a).

The workshop "Adventures in Voice" (AIV), also developed and presented by Katherine Verdolini Abbott, adapts the principles of individualized treatment along the Voice Therapy Spectrum to the pediatric population. The AIV program is designed for children with voice disorders associated with hypo- or hyperadduction of the vocal folds. This functional disorder encompasses the majority of children seen for voice therapy. The AIV program works with the natural phonatory behaviors of children, rather than restricting behaviors. For example, traditional approaches attempt to restrict shouting in children with voice disorders. AIV teaches children how to shout in a manner that will not be as vocally abusive. This perspective is based on theories regarding the intrinsically rewarding nature of "fun" activities, such as practicing vocally healthy shouting, and the potential for intrinsic motivation to boost compliance and ultimately increase gains in vocal health (Verdolini Abbott, 2012b).

The Accent Method was developed by Svend Smith in Denmark many years ago. Kotby, Shiromoto, and Hirano (1993) have outlined a procedure for the method and documented its effect on the voice through therapy procedures. The Accent Method targets voice weakness by developing abdominal breathing for supported phonation and coordinating motion of the vocal folds, the articulators, and the entire body for efficient speech production (Stemple et al., 2010). The procedure for the Accent Method is divided into exercises targeting respiration, vocal function, and speech. The clinician begins by instructing the child in an abdominal breathing pattern that will facilitate phonation. Once this pattern has been established, the child begins vocal exercises wherein she produces soft, breathy phonation while making a fricative (s, sh, f) or a closed vowel sound (high vowels /i/ or /u/). After sustaining each sound individually, a two-beat rhythm is accented, with the first sound produced weakly and the second sound more forcefully and sustained, such as "s-S---------". This is followed by any combination of consonants and vowels ("ba" or "you"). The child progresses through the exercises at different tempos: largo (slow), andante (moderate), and allegro (fast). Arm movements, tapping, or a drum can be used to establish these tempos during the exercises. The number of syllables and syllable stress are modified within each tempo. When performing the exercises within the largo tempo, the child places stress on one or two syllables in a phrase ("ba-BA" or "ba-BA-BA"). Andante exercises include three stressed syllables ("ba-BA-BA-BA) and allegro exercises require five

stressed syllables ("ba-BA-BA-BA-BA-BA"). The final procedure is transferring the rhythm and stress to oral reading with marked phrases, followed by conversation. This method is often employed for vocal professionals and has been used to treat fluency disorders (Moller, 2006). Children who enjoy singing and rhythmical activities can relate to the structure of the Accent Method.

Adapting Adult Techniques for Children/Improving Compliance

Voice Aerobics™ is an exercise program that incorporates VFEs with light physical activity and is designed to be administered three times a week. The exercise DVDs were developed and are distributed by Mary Spremulli, speech-language pathologist, for individuals who have lost vocal power and range. Originally designed for patients with Parkinson disease, the DVDs are geared toward an older patient population (Spremulli, 2008). However, the concept of combining vocal exercise with kinesthetic movement could be adapted for children in creative ways that might boost engagement and compliance with therapy.

Regardless of the treatment techniques used in voice therapy, an important consideration is to evaluate the feelings and personality of the children. Comment upon their positive behaviors to encourage participation and willingness to perform the tasks necessary for resolution of the voice disorder. If there are underlying personality issues that curtail compliance, these will need to be addressed with the child and family.

Child and Adolescent Differences

Children and adolescents may have similarities, but they also have differences. Younger children may have more of a desire to please the authority figure compared with adolescents. Children are more willing to accept support from an adult, whereas the adolescents seek more independence. Extrinsic rewards are more effective with children compared with intrinsic reinforcement for adolescents. Parents are typically more involved in homework assignments with children versus adolescents. Children require longer time periods for practicing skills, whereas adolescents need to be counseled to accept the concepts of the voice treatment as applicable to their lifestyle (Andrews, 2002).

Technology and Therapy

Technology has provided a plethora of opportunities to facilitate healthy voice use on a daily basis. Voice amplification devices, such as ChatterVox®, have been available for a number of years for individuals who have difficulty projecting their voice (e.g., due to vocal fold paralysis) or require a reduction in "vocal dose" (e.g., due to hyperadduction of the vocal folds with frequent excessive loudness). For the purposes of monitoring voice use, the Ambulatory Phonation Monitor (APM; Model 3200; KayPENTAX) is a portable device that records how individuals use their voices throughout the day. The APM can also expedite carryover of therapy goals outside the clinical environment via the use of real-time vibrotactile feedback.

The use of gaming and apps in pediatric voice therapy brings exciting new possibilities for motivating children during treatment. Many children encounter technology daily in their homes and at school and expect the kind of individualization and visual stimulation that this type of technology can provide. Some of the feedback provided by this technology immediately illustrates for children

which of their voicing behaviors are successful and which are undesirable and potentially harmful.

Gaming

There are many gaming options available for use in voice therapy, particularly for children. KayPENTAX (Montvale, NJ) has a variety of Voice Games (Model 5167B) for use with their software, such as Visi-Pitch IV (Model 3950; KayPENTAX; Instruction Manual Issue F, 2009). They provide an animated, real-time, graphic approach to treatment of speech and voice parameters. Available games address phonation duration, frequency or amplitude control, frequency or amplitude range, frequency or amplitude modulation, and voicing (on/off). These games are categorized based on their ability to address the various voice parameters.

For children with poor breath support, three Voice Games are the Monkey game, the Croaker game, and the Frog Hop game (Figure 6–1). All three games allow the clinician to control the number of trials and the level of

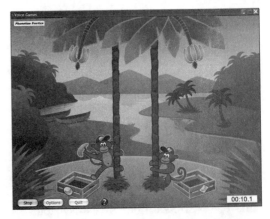

Figure 6–1. Voice Games—Phonation Practice. Courtesy of KayPENTAX.

difficulty of the stimulus. The Monkey game and the Croaker game elicit sustained phonation by providing a reward for increased duration of phonation. For example, the clinician sets a duration interval of 1 to 10 seconds in the Croaker game. An interval of 2 requires 2 seconds of phonation for a reward. The child produces a voiced/unvoiced "papapa" sequence for the selected interval. As the child's duration of phonation increases, the throat of an animated frog grows until it emits a fun "croaking" sound. The child then "collects" this frog and either finishes the game or continues to the interval when 10 frogs have been collected. The silly sounds and images are rewarding and engaging while providing meaningful feedback about the child's vocal performance (KayPENTAX; Instruction Manual Issue F, 2009).

The Frog Hop game also helps a child improve voice onset time. The clinician selects a level of difficulty for the child, which adjusts the speed of the game. The goal of the game is to cause a frog to jump from one lily pad to another to reach a destination in a river. The lily pads move in the water. The child's vocalization causes the frog to jump from one lily pad to another, but the frog does so only when voicing is detected by the software. Therefore, the child must time his voice onset precisely, for if he begins voicing too early or too late, his frog will miss the lily pad and fall into the water. Again, children can interact with the game independently and have immediate visual feedback about their voice onset time. This is engaging and motivating for the child. The difficulty of the task can grow with the child's abilities. Adolescents may even select the level of difficulty for themselves, encouraging self-awareness of their own abilities and helping them to assume an active, responsible role during their therapy session (KayPENTAX Instruction Manual Issue F, 2009).

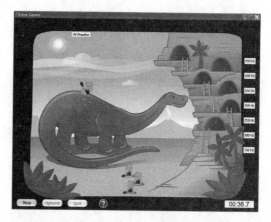

Figure 6–2. Voice Games—F_0 Practice. Courtesy of KayPENTAX.

Other games address pitch and loudness. The Dinosaur Slide game can address pitch range, pitch modulation, pitch duration, easy amplitude onset, and phonation duration (Figure 6–2). The clinician selects a level of difficulty that decreases or increases the length of the stimulus. The clinician also enters minimum and maximum target ranges for fundamental frequency and/or amplitude. As the child phonates into the microphone, the dinosaur's head moves closer to a caveman when the desired amplitude and/or pitch are produced. The child "wins" the game after a certain number of cavemen have hopped onto the dinosaur's head and slid down its back. The game allows for clinician control over the child's target fundamental frequency and amplitude ranges, aiding in the process of shaping the child toward improved phonation. The game Dragon Blast operates in a similar manner (Figure 6–3, KayPENTAX Instruction Manual Issue F, 2009).

Penguin Party, as well as other games with similar controls and objectives, can be used with children working on pitch control, pitch range, inappropriate pitch, monotone pitch, pitch modulation, and inappropriate loudness. The object of the game is for the

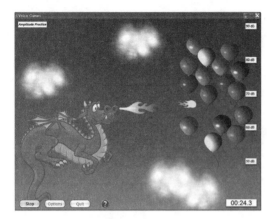

Figure 6–3. Voice Games—Amplitude Practice. Courtesy of KayPENTAX.

child to guide a penguin from one side of the screen to the other while using phonation modulation to avoid obstacles (icebergs). The clinician can vary the speed at which the penguin travels across the screen, number of trials, and level of difficulty of the obstacle placement. The clinician also specifies the target fundamental frequency and/or amplitude for the child. By staying within the specified range, the child successfully guides the penguin. Other forms of this game involve fishing, guiding a butterfly to flowers, and helping a dragon to pop balloons with his flaming breath. The various versions allow children to develop a "favorite" game (KayPENTAX Instruction Manual Issue F, 2009).

King, Davis, Lehman, and Ruddy (2012) demonstrated that a video game designed for entertainment could be modified for voice treatment and utilized to motivate children to practice therapy techniques both in treatment sessions and at home. In this study, researchers analyzed a solely entertainment-based, competitive computer game called *Opera Slinger* 1.0 (Treblemakers, Florida Interactive Entertainment Academy at the University of Central Florida, Orlando) through three levels of feasibility testing. The game was modified fol-

lowing each level of testing in an effort to tailor the game for use as a therapeutic procedure. During the third level of testing, a 9-year-old male with a diagnosis of hyperfunctional voice disorder utilized the game during his second phase of voice treatment. The date, time, and frequency of exercises were recorded daily. The participant's mother reported that her son was highly motivated to complete the levels of the game repeatedly without being instructed to do so at home.

Apps for Google Android and Apple iOS Devices

An increasing number of SLPs are beginning to implement the use of applications (apps) in their communication therapy sessions. While many of the SLP-friendly apps that are currently available focus on articulation and forms of augmentative and alternative communication (AAC), a variety of apps have been introduced that are specifically related to voice therapy or may be adapted for voice treatment with both adult and pediatric patients (Figure 6–4). The following information regarding voice applications is a summary of a professional workshop presentation (Maira, Hapner, & Olson, 2012). All of the applications mentioned in this review were available at the time of this publication with free trial versions or within the price range of $.99 to $2.34. The reviewed applications are available for Android devices (Google), iOS devices (Apple), or both.

When utilizing some pediatric voice treatments, such as VFEs, the child's pitch range must be determined and the clinician must provide an appropriate musical note for the child to imitate. The Android application *DaTuner* (Applaud Apps) serves as both a pitch-pipe and a tuner. When utilizing the app in therapy, the color of the digit

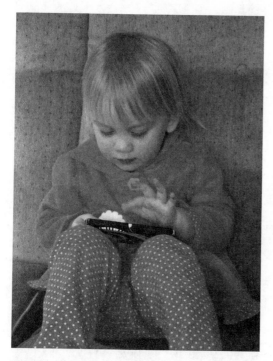

Figure 6–4. Young child playing a game on a mobile device.

display changes to green once the reading is in tune. An additional Android app that may be utilized as both a tuner and pitch-pipe is *G-Strings* (cohortor.org). This application was designed to serve as a chromatic tuner for violins, guitars, and other instruments. The application provides real-time pitch assessment and is additionally beneficial for immediate biofeedback. Apps that provide scales for vocal warm-up include *Piano DX* (Better Day Wireless) and *Mobile Warm-Ups* (Goodman Productions) for iOS devices.

In addition to applications for pitch settings, apps have been developed to measure loudness and encourage vocal rest. There are several applications available that function as sound level meters. The *Decibel Meter* (TA-COTY CN) application for Android devices operates as a sound level meter with analog and digital feedback, as well as a method of

calibration. A similar application called *Digital Sound Meter Free* (Patrick Giudicelli) has been created for iOS devices. Especially when working with young children, it can become difficult to encourage vocal rest. Applications such as *iSpeech* (Orange Driver Software) and *Speak It* (Future Apps) have been designed for iOS devices and serve as text-to-speech options that can be recommended to children and their parents for use at home while on voice rest (Figure 6–5). *Air Horn* (Simpaddico) is an additional application created for both iOS and Android devices that performs as a noisemaker. If families have access to a device for home use, clinicians can encourage children to utilize the app as an alternative to shouting throughout the house. *Voice Changer Plus* (Art Software) is an additional application that was created for iOS devices and can record a child's voice and replay it in a variety of formats. The child's voice can be played back louder to encourage the child to use the app rather than raising his or her voice in loud environments. To record audio or video footage from a session, applications such as *iTalk* (Griffin Technology) for iOS and *Vimeo* (Vimeo) for both iOS and Android may be utilized. Additionally, drawing applications such as *Drawing Pad* (Darren Murtha Design)

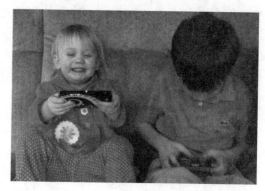

Figure 6–5. Children using mobile devices for gaming and apps.

for both iOS and Android devices allow the user to draw with a large variety of markers, crayons, colored pencils, paints, and chalks for reinforcement during therapy or for the clinician to illustrate processes of respiration, phonation, and resonance for pediatric patients.

There are many game applications available on iOS and Android devices that may be adapted for pediatric voice treatment. *Talking Tom Cat 2* is a free iOS and Android application featuring a cat character that repeats the speaker's voice in a high-pitch format. This can be motivating and fun for children, and it can increase their awareness of personal vocal roughness (Figure 6–6). The application was created by Out Fit 7, which also offers applications featuring many other characters that provide voice playback in silly voices.

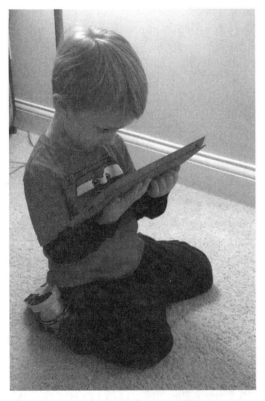

Figure 6–6. Young boy using tablet device.

Telehealth and Pediatric Voice Therapy

In recent years, telehealth has emerged as an option for providing speech-language services to those who have difficulty accessing care due to geography or are in areas severely underserved by clinicians. Beijer, Rietveld, Hoskam, Geurts, and de Swart (2009) showed that an independent e-learning program for those with dysarthria resulting from Parkinson disease did increase intelligibility in connected speech and showed patient satisfaction with the model. Constintanescu and colleagues (2011) also documented patient satisfaction with the telehealth model. This study compared two groups undergoing a patented speech and voice treatment program, the Lee Silverman Voice Treatment®. One group received instruction in person and the other group completed the program through online sessions. Both groups benefited similarly from the program, with no documented disadvantage for the group receiving online treatment (Constintanescu et al., 2011).

Current evidence considers telehealth for adults, but what are the uses of telehealth for the treatment of children? Although the research in this area is limited, the success of telehealth for improving families' access to SLPs for the treatment of pediatric speech and language disorders has been documented. Grogan-Johnson, Alvares, Rowan, and Creaghead (2010) conducted a pediatric study in rural Ohio similar to that of Constintanescu and colleagues (2011) with adults. Grogan-Johnson and researchers implemented the same speech-language therapy program in two school systems, one via face-to-face therapy and the other with telehealth methods. Over a period of 4 months, the telehealth clinicians in these rural areas videoconferenced with subjects while they were at school. An "e-helper" stationed at the school helped to facilitate the session, as well as set up and troubleshoot the technology. When the study concluded, results showed no difference in therapy outcomes between the students who received service through telehealth and those who had face-to-face interaction with the clinicians. Furthermore, those in the telehealth group reported being satisfied or extremely satisfied with the experience (Grogan-Johnson et al.).

Because most frequently occurring pediatric voice disorders (e.g., nodules) typically do not co-occur with other complex communication disorders, the potential benefit of telehealth service in this discrete category of pediatric voice disorder is high. There are also obvious economic benefits that result from the efficiency with which treatment can be distributed. Additionally, the use of telehealth can reduce the burden of travel for SLPs whose service area is geographically great.

Questions about the use of telehealth exist, including concerns about its logistical details (e.g., the impact of technical issues on the session). Also, some question the impact of decreased face-to-face time for clinician interaction and the implications for patient feedback and individualized treatment. While telehealth has the potential to link SLPs with pediatric voice specialty to those who might not otherwise have access to such a professional due to geographic location, more research is needed regarding the development and implementation of telehealth for treatment of pediatric voice disorders.

> ### Pediatric Performer: Considerations for Performing Voice—Childhood Through Adolescence

Contributed by Wendy LeBorgne

Understanding the pediatric and adolescent performing voice warrants unique consider-

ation. Although children begin singing/imitating songs and melodic variations they hear at a young age, it is often their exposure to vocal music in a choral situation (church, school, or community) that sparks an interest for further voice training. Also, occasionally parents actively pursue vocal training for their child, hoping to generate the next "star." Within the current pop culture, children and parents are inundated with unrealistic expectations of what young girls and boys should sound like, without a full understanding of the demands placed on this type of performance and the potential injury-risk associated with it. Young professional vocal athletes are similar to elite Olympic gymnasts, and issues related to their physical, emotional, and cognitive development must be understood by voice professionals who prevent, evaluate, and treat vocal injury in this population. This section of the text outlines historical pedagogical training of young voices, age/development-specific considerations, and concerns for vocal injury within this subset of performers.

Historical Vocal Pedagogy of Young Singers

The "appropriate age" for a child to begin vocal training remains controversial in the singing community. Historically, voice teachers have debated the minimum age to begin private vocal training. Some teachers believe that no child is too young to begin training, while others believe that training should not begin until after puberty. The American Academy of Teachers of Singing endorsed training young voices by qualified voice teachers in 2002. Boychoir singing (within the church) may be some of the earliest professional youth vocal performances and dates back to the late Middle Ages in the Viennese Court. Vocal prodigies have been present throughout the centuries, just as any athletes, but with today's popular media culture, very young child performers are often exploited for their talents. Parents seek out vocal teachers to train young voices often without knowledge or understanding of technical voice training.

There are multiple possibilities for exposing a young child to vocal music without enrollment in an intensive vocal training program. Musical stimulation in children should be encouraged, but never forced. Parents of preschool-aged children should encourage their child to sing along with music from shows such as *Sesame Street* and *Veggie Tales*. Organized music programs that specifically target children, such as Kinder-music, are excellent resources for introducing music appreciation and ear training to infants and toddlers. In addition, many churches begin children's choirs as early as age 3 years. Choral singing in a group environment provides young children an outlet to sing with others their age (Atkinson, 2010; Hook, 1998; Phillips, 1992; Rutkowski & Miller, 2002; Siupsinskiene & Lycke, 2011; Welch, 1988). These types of venues provide age-appropriate music and are typically limited in vocal range and musical complexity. School-age children are exposed to vocal music as part of the school's curriculum. Music education in the schools typically involves both vocal and instrumental training. A child's participation in choirs and/or musical presentations is often a young singer's first exposure to public performance. If a child of elementary school age demonstrates an aptitude and eagerness to further engage in singing, one may consider private or group lessons. Professional children's choirs can provide children the opportunity to learn good vocal technique in a group situation. Community and professional theater productions often have roles for children. The classical singing world has generally more limited roles for children, but the Metropolitan Opera maintains an active

children's vocal program where students in the program are used in choral and solo roles.

Unlike SLPs or music educators within the educational system, there is no formal certification or education required to become a private vocal instructor. Historically, vocal pedagogues worked in a master/apprentice relationship. In order to be considered for acceptance into a given vocal studio, the student had to pass a rigorous audition process that included natural vocal talent, good looks, willingness/ability to train, commitment to training, and a lack of vocal flaws (Appelman, 1967; Miller, 1996, 2000, 2009; Sataloff, 1998; Vennard, 1967). Once a student was accepted into a studio, he faced a 2- to 5-year process of vocal training, working only on technique: No songs were allowed to be sung, he worked on only vocal exercises. Students were expected to be committed to daily vocal practice and adequately care for their vocal instrument and body. Furthermore, if they did not follow the directions of their teacher (or did not make expected vocal progress), they were dismissed from the vocal studio.

Today's vocal training programs are often financially driven and if a student is paying for voice lessons, a product (recital, performance, etc.) is typically expected within 3 months of initiating vocal training. This model may not provide enough basic vocal training for the pliable laryngeal musculature to develop appropriate motor patterns. Training neuromuscular patterns requires drill and repetition. Vocal drills (called vocalises) to train agility and flexibility should be fun and creative for young voices and thus encourage a willingness to engage in daily practice. There is preliminary scientific evidence documenting the efficacy of singing voice training for prepubescent and pubescent voices (Andrews, 1997; Barlow & Howard, 2002, 2005; Blatt, 1983; Bonet & Casan, 1994; Cornut, Riou-Bourret, & Louis, 1971; Edwin, 1997;

Lundy, Roy, Casiano, Xue, & Evans, 2000; Reilly, 1995; Schneider, Zumtobel, Prettenhofer, Aichstill, & Jocher, 2010; Siupsinskiene & Lycke, 2011; Skelton, 2007). Private instruction for the truly interested and talented child should include education regarding appropriate vocal hygiene, experimentation with high and low sounds (within a limited range), experimentation with loud and soft singing (within a musically acceptable range), and appropriate breathing techniques. When seeking private vocal instruction, good teachers and studios should provide an initial consultation visit in order to determine whether a child is ready for voice lessons physically, emotionally, and musically. Repertoire for the young child should be age and voice range appropriate and should be emotionally within his or her present life experiences.

One current pedagogical approach to training children's voices is for the singing teacher to take on the role of "vocal parent." Edwin (1995, 1997, 2001) advocates singing with different colors to help the child experiment with timbre (e.g., "sing a hot pink /i/," "sing a navy blue /u/"). One game, called the Human Boom Box, teaches children to alter timbre by having them "turn up the treble" or "boost the bass" in their voices. Ideally, these exercises will teach the vocal students that they are capable of producing many different vocal sounds. It then becomes the goal of the voice teacher to influence the child's perception of good singing by maintaining a balanced, even vocal production throughout the vocal range. Providing good vocal models in the studio and suggesting appropriate role models in the "pop" culture and classical world will also help to influence young singers in a positive way.

Many young vocal students successfully emulate the vocal style of unhealthy vocal techniques (hard glottal attacks, breathy voices, glottal fry phonation, and singing too

high or out of range) demonstrated in the pop world. In some popular singing styles, dysphonia is considered a desired quality. Individuals with unique voices (not always perfectly healthy) get hired. Vocal professionals should strive to promote a healthy, efficient singing voice, with adequate agility and flexibility in the musculature to perform various vocal tasks with ease, in order to minimize/prevent injury.

Considerations for Singing During Puberty

Vocal training during puberty is an additional source of controversy among singing teachers, and the pedagogical literature on vocal training during puberty is mixed (Brown, 1996; Sataloff, 1998). Improved scientific understanding of the physiologic and acoustic developmental markers during puberty may provide a basis for improved research in the area of vocal training through puberty (Boltezar, Burger, & Zargi, 1997; Boseley & Hartnick, 2006; Dejonckere, Wieneke, Bloemenkamp, & LeBacq, 1996; Fatterpekar, Mukherji, Rajgopalan, Lin, & Castillo, 2004; Fitch & Giedd, 1999; Hartnick & Boseley, 2008; Hartnick, Rehbar, & Prasad, 2005; Hasek, Singh, & Murry, 1980; Kahane, 1978; McAllister & Sundberg, 1998; McAllister, Sederholm, Sundberg, & Gramming, 1994; Mecke & Sundberg, 2010; Reilly, 1995; Sergeant & Welch, 2009; Trollinger, 2007; Whiteside, Hodgson, & Tapster, 2002; Yarnell, 2006). If the adolescent performer is singing in a public or professional arena, the voice teacher can provide insight, education, and reassurance to the singer, who is experiencing a significant vocal transformation. The voice pathologist or singing teacher may alleviate anxiety through education on physiological laryngeal changes that occur during puberty. With male students, discussion regarding the often drastic and audible vocal change may be beneficial. Research on the implications of male adolescent voice change has been well documented by many studies involving members of boy-choir ensembles (Collins, 2006; Cooksey, 1999; Friar, 1999; Hollien, 2011; Killian, 1999; McKenzie, 1956; Pedersen, Møller, Krabbe, Munk, & Bennett, 1985; Skadsem, 2007; Swanson, 1984; Williams, Welch, & Howard, 2005). Similarly, female students should be made aware of vocal changes that may occur around their menstrual cycle and hormone fluctuations (Abitbol, Abitbol, & Abitbol, 1999; Cooksey, 1999; Decoster, Ghesquiere, & Van Steenberge, 2008; Echternach et al., 2010; Williams, Larson, & Price, 1996). An attempt to answer all questions parents and adolescents may pose regarding pubescent voice change requires an understanding of the laryngeal physiologic maturation process.

If a singer plans (or is required) to continue singing during puberty, general parameters for ongoing vocal training are warranted. First, heavy voice use during vocal mutation should be avoided. For the professional adolescent singer (specifically males), this may mean taking 6 months to a year off from a heavy performance schedule. Second, the endurance of the vocal mechanism may be limited. Therefore, voice lessons should never last longer than a half hour, and practice sessions should be short in duration (15 minutes, twice a day). Third, all singing should be done in a comfortable mid-range at a medium vocal intensity level. This comfortable range may vary from week to week or even day to day, especially in the male voice. With an esteemed singer/teacher/voice pathologist relationship, adolescent singers should learn to respect and identify their comfortable voice during puberty.

In addition to the above-mentioned considerations for the adolescent voice, a special mention regarding the young, breathy female voice is in order. A breathy vocal quality is often considered a vocal flaw in a professional singer. However, breathy voices, especially in young females, are typical and have been shown to increase in the degree of breathiness following the onset of menstruation (Miller, 1995; Williams, Larson, & Price, 1996). The breathy vocal quality exhibited by young female singers is typically the result of a large posterior glottis gap in conjunction with discoordination of the muscles of respiration, phonation, and resonance. If a voice teacher attempts to eliminate all of the normal breathiness by increasing vocal fold adduction in a forced manner, it may have long-term detrimental effects on the voice by creating laryngeal hyperfunction. The voice pathologist must be able to distinguish the difference in breathiness and hoarseness, especially at high frequency phonation.

Singing through adolescence without vocal difficulty is possible if appropriate considerations regarding the mutational voice change are followed. Lee, Pennington, and Stemple (1998) completed a study that lends support to private vocal study for high school students who are active performers. They examined eight high school leads in a musical theater production, pre-rehearsal and post-performance. No vocal disorders were found among this group of singers at pre-rehearsal or post-performance. All of the leads in this study had at least one year of private vocal instruction, and they were double cast, requiring a decreased (and manageable) amount of performance time. These findings suggested that if the vocal demands of a young singer are reasonable (double casting) and if appropriate singing techniques are employed (private training), then they may maintain a healthy laryngeal mechanism.

Pedagogical debates regarding training of the adolescent voice will continue to persist in the voice community until empirical studies document the efficacy of specific training modalities. Vocal training must include adequate comprehension about the nature and function of the laryngeal mechanism. Specifically, physical, cognitive, emotional, and musical abilities must be realistically assessed in each child. This assessment should provide the basis for early vocal training with the understanding that each child must be trained on an individual basis with techniques appropriate for the young and changing voice. Empirical studies documenting the efficacy of vocal training continue to be warranted.

Laryngeal Pathology in the Pediatric Performer

Unlike the literature available on the physiologic, anthropometric, and psychological development and understanding of young elite physical athletes, which provides insight into injury prevention and treatment, there are limited studies regarding parallel parameters in young vocal athletes (Benninger, 2011; Reilly, 1995; Verduyckt, Remacle, Jamart, Benderitter, & Morsomme, 2011). Therefore, the research on vocal injury within the professional singing population is limited primarily to the late adolescent, college student, and adult populations (Tepe et al., 2002). Similar to perceptual assessment in the adult, dysphonia, loss of frequency range, throat pain, resonance abnormalities, or any abnormal vocal symptom in the young singer warrants a referral to an otolaryngologist to rule out any possible laryngeal pathology. A voice pathologist's assessment of aerodynamic, acoustic, and stroboscopic parameters is also warranted to note subtle changes in mucosal flexibility, glottic closure patterns, and so forth. Also, a technical voice assessment may be vital for a complete understanding of the impact of the vocal problem and provision of adequate treatment planning. When investigating the vocal dif-

ficulties of young choral performers (ages 3–25 years), Tepe and colleagues noted that 55.8% reported some vocal problem, and the late adolescent was most at risk for vocal difficulty. Research studies that provide preliminary insights into common vocal pathologies of professional voice users include overuse injuries, vocal fold lesions from phonotraumatic behaviors, and reflux. However, pediatric vocal performers cannot be considered small adult performers, and the majority of the literature regarding habits and injuries cannot be transferred without adequate scientific evidence.

Pulling It All Together: Case Summaries

The following seven cases represent children who presented with a variety of voice disorders. Each case summary is written with a brief history, voice evaluation, summary of treatment procedures, and treatment outcomes. The treatment procedures employed with these cases have been discussed within this chapter.

Case 1. Patient: Lancer (Bilateral Vocal Fold Lesions)

History

Lancer was an 8-year-old male with a history of intermittent dysphonia. His additional, pertinent history included asthma, seasonal allergies, and an articulation disorder, for which he was receiving speech therapy. The episodes of dysphonia had been noted for several years and the onset was always following a cold or asthma attack. Most recently, Lancer had experienced an episode of dysphonia that did not resolve, and the episode's onset was not following a cold or asthma attack. Lancer's clinician had noticed the intermittent occurrences of his chronic dysphonia during speech therapy sessions. Therefore, Lancer was subsequently referred for a comprehensive voice evaluation.

Voice Evaluation

At his initial voice evaluation, Lancer presented with moderate-to-severe dysphonia characterized primarily by increased strain, but also roughness, pitch breaks, and limited pitch range. A flexible stroboscopic examination revealed bilateral vocal fold lesions. The right vocal fold lesion appeared slightly larger and more rounded, while the left lesion appeared broad based. The child's family expressed that they were not interested in the surgical excision of Lancer's vocal fold lesions. Recommendations included voice therapy, with follow-up voice evaluation and stroboscopic examination in 3 to 4 months after a course of voice therapy was completed.

Summary of the Treatment Procedures

An SLP, who was able to administer voice therapy in combination with the articulation therapy that Lancer still needed, initiated the treatment. The voice treatment procedure included vocal hygiene, VFEs, and resonance therapy. Vocal hygiene aspects included reducing phonotraumatic behaviors and increasing hydration. Lancer frequently used a loud voice and yelled in his daily activities. VFEs were initiated first, followed by the addition of resonance therapy. The treatment procedure additionally focused on reducing laryngeal strain and tension. Lancer and his family were very compliant with voice therapy and they adequately completed the associated voice therapy tasks at home during the 3-month treatment period. Due to his musical background, Lancer demonstrated particular strengths in pitch matching during both VFEs and resonance therapy, and did not require much adaptation of these exercises from the format used with adults. Lancer demonstrated increased maximum phonation times for the VFEs and progressed through Step 5 with resonance therapy.

Treatment Outcomes

After 3 months, a posttherapy voice evaluation was completed. At this evaluation, Lancer presented with mild to moderate dysphonia characterized by strain and roughness. Perceptual voice quality was improved in comparison with his initial voice evaluation, and reduced strain was particularly noted. A flexible stroboscopic examination revealed persistent vocal fold lesions, with the right lesion still appearing larger than the left. Hourglass glottic closure was observed; however, closure was improved in comparison with the initial voice evaluation. Improved perceptual voice quality and increased maximum phonation times had occurred over the past 3 months, and Lancer's progress had not yet plateaued. Therefore, it was recommended that he continue voice therapy and return to the voice clinic 6 months later for reassessment of his vocal fold lesions.

Lancer continued to receive both voice and articulation therapy. The voice therapy portion of his sessions consisted of completing the resonance therapy program, maintaining improved perceptual voice, and continuing both VFEs and resonance therapy as a home program. A portion of the session was spent recording VFEs each week, and Lancer continued to demonstrate increased maximum phonation times. Lancer and his family were consistently compliant with completing the voice therapy tasks at home. Perceptual voice quality continued to improve, and phonotrauma decreased across all environments.

At the 6-month follow-up voice evaluation, Lancer presented with only mild dysphonia characterized by strain and roughness. A comparison of acoustic samples revealed significant perceptual voice improvement. Although a flexible stroboscopic examination revealed persistent bilateral vocal fold lesions, particular improvement with vocal fold flexibility and glottic closure was noted. Lancer and his family noticed perceptual voice improvement and did not express any further concern regarding his voice. Due to persistent articulation errors and difficulty with carryover of speech sounds to connected speech, Lancer continued to receive articulation therapy. A follow-up visit to the voice clinic was recommended for one year to complete a routine examination of the vocal folds.

Case 2. Patient: Tom (Bilateral Vocal Fold Lesions)

History

Tom was a 9-year-old male who was seen in the voice clinic for an evaluation of dysphonia. His history included an onset of hoarseness that his family began noticing 10 weeks prior. It was reported that Tom engaged in loud talking, especially during sports.

Voice Evaluation

Tom's voice evaluation revealed moderate to severe dysphonia characterized by roughness, strain, low pitch for his age and gender, and periods of aphonia. A stroboscopic examination revealed large, bilateral vocal fold lesions, with the right lesion larger than the left. During phonation, incomplete glottic closure was observed with mild supraglottic compression. The source of phonation was the patient's true vocal folds. Surgery for removal of the

vocal fold lesions was discussed as a possibility after completing 8 weeks of therapy.

Summary of the Treatment Procedures

Voice therapy techniques included VFEs, resonance therapy, and vocal hygiene. These techniques were chosen to help reduce supraglottic tension, promote healthier vocal fold vibration, and improve focus on breath support when the patient needed to yell during sports. Modifications were made to the direct treatment techniques due to Tom's ability to perform the exercises. Activities included nasal /ee/ on comfortable pitch; glide up; glide down; low, comfortable, and high pitch /ol/; phrases and sentences with nasal consonants; and phrases and sentences with varied consonants.

Treatment Outcomes

Five therapy sessions were completed prior to the follow-up voice evaluation. Audio samples revealed voice quality improvement; however, the stroboscopic examination showed the continued presence of vocal fold lesions, although the size had diminished. The family decided to proceed with surgery. Five days postsurgery with complete vocal rest, an endoscopic examination revealed significant healing. Tom was instructed to use his voice only when needed, not play sports at this time, and return for voice therapy. When Tom was seen for his first session, he had continued to improve. Tom was instructed to begin using his voice minimally. During his second voice therapy visit, there was a significant increase in roughness. He returned to the voice clinic, and a stroboscopic examination revealed a large unilateral lesion. At that time, he was placed on voice rest for 2 weeks. When he returned to the voice clinic, the lesion had decreased in size, but it was still prominent. Therefore, he returned to the operating room, and the otolaryngologist injected a steroid and placed Tom on prescribed steroids. One week post-injection with complete vocal rest, an examination showed a significant decrease in lesion size. Tom was instructed to continue voice therapy and follow up in the voice clinic in 3 months. Tom was seen one or two times per month for voice therapy during this time and he demonstrated consistent improvement. His 3-month follow-up visit continued to reveal an improved lesion site. The child and his family were happy with the results and he was scheduled to be seen at the voice clinic in 6 to 12 months.

Case 3. Patient: Elizabeth (Functional Voice Loss)

History

Elizabeth was a 16-year-old female who experienced laryngitis secondary to an upper respiratory illness. Her voice loss remained after the illness had resolved. She saw an otolaryngologist, who diagnosed a functional voice loss, telling her she needed to "relearn to use her voice." Reportedly, she sought the services of her school-based SLP without improvement. She remained aphonic for 7 months, until she received her school schedule for the upcoming year and noted that "choir" was one of the classes listed. She knew that she would need a functional voice in order to participate in that course.

Voice Evaluation

Elizabeth was seen for a voice evaluation, which revealed significant vocal strain, with only a forced whisper being produced. Using visual feedback via the KayPENTAX Visi Pitch IV software program, she was able to produce voicing, although it remained very strained and high pitched.

Summary of the Treatment Procedures

Elizabeth was seen for voice therapy, with emphasis on using a forward focus voice and visual feedback (Visi-Pitch IV). During the second session, she produced a more relaxed voice with appropriate pitch, which began to carry over into conversational speech throughout the session. Elizabeth returned for her next session without any progress noted. She expressed some worry about using her voice outside of the treatment room. Therefore, therapy was moved into the hallway, and although she was able to demonstrate use of her voice in that environment, she reverted to a whisper when someone walked by. The structure of therapy was then geared toward desensitization, such as using her voice in the elevator or speaking to the SLP in the presence of an unknown person, which she successfully achieved during the third session. Elizabeth then expressed a desire to "show" her voice to her mother and sister, who had accompanied her to the session. They entered the therapy room and with a slight hesitation Elizabeth was able to voice. However, during the following week, she was not able to use her voice at home with her mother and her sister. This was set as a goal, which she achieved by the fourth session. However, she had not yet used her voice at school or with her father.

Treatment Outcomes

Elizabeth seemed "stuck" for 2 weeks, until she suddenly came in for her sixth session and reported that she had "shown" her best friend her voice. She was able to successfully use her voice in the classroom and with her peers by her seventh session. On her last therapy session, she came in to say that she had attempted to "show" her voice to her father. However, when she approached him, he "shooed" her away, due to his involvement in some other task. Her mother explained Elizabeth's intent and Elizabeth then "showed" her father her voice, at which time he began to cry. As she retold this story to the SLP, she stated, "I didn't know he loved me this much." Although Elizabeth and her mother had been reluctant to pursue psychotherapy, it was evident that there were some emotional issues. Most concerning was the fact that the family had not pursued active voice therapy outside of the school until 7 months after Elizabeth had lost her voice. It was conjectured that Elizabeth's initial voice loss due to her illness provided her with the opportunity to escape some of the verbal interactions with her family, and it became habituated.

Case 4. Patient: Audrey (Anterior Laryngeal Web and Chronic High Pitch Voice)

History

Audrey was an 11-year-old female with a history of anterior laryngeal web and a chronic high-pitched voice that had been noted by the family over the past several years. Audrey's family reported that when she was younger her voice sounded higher in pitch than her same-age peers. However, it was only over the past several years, as Audrey became older, that her high-pitched voice had become more problematic. Several months prior to this evaluation, Audrey underwent an initial surgical division of her anterior laryngeal web. Although initial voice improvement was noted following surgery, perceptual voice quality (higher pitch) returned to baseline as the web reformed.

Voice Evaluation

Audrey was referred for a voice evaluation and presented with moderate to severe dysphonia characterized by high pitch, breathiness, de-creased volume, and roughness. An anterior laryngeal web was noted, and only the posterior one-third segment of the true vocal folds demonstrated vibratory movement. Following a second surgical division of the anterior laryngeal web, Audrey presented with decreased pitch during sustained phonation tasks. With trial voice therapy tasks, Audrey was able to decrease her pitch even further toward an age-appropriate level. Voice therapy was then initiated.

Summary of the Treatment Procedures

Audrey's voice therapy goals focused on decreasing fundamental frequency and increasing vocal volume. She had developed a pattern of high-pitched voice, strain, and breathiness that persisted after the surgical division of her anterior laryngeal web. Audrey received voice therapy for 3 months. Therapy sessions initially consisted of completing VFEs and resonance therapy tasks. During therapy sessions, time was spent distinguishing between high, medium, and low pitch levels. Audrey was immediately able to distinguish between these pitches; however, she demonstrated difficulty matching them. Pitches for the power-building portion of the VFEs initially consisted of three notes that were slightly higher than the norm for Audrey's age. Lower pitches were gradually introduced, and Audrey was eventually able to complete VFEs within the C4 to G4 range, which was typical for Audrey's age. Using a forward focus gesture, including a lip buzz to "glide" from a higher to a lower pitch and then sustain the lower pitch was quite effective for eliciting lower pitches. Audrey demonstrated a consistent increase in maximum phonation times for VFEs during the first 2 months, and then she plateaued. VFEs were beneficial for eliciting and distinguishing appropriate pitch, with an engaging, forward focus voice in order to decrease breathiness and increase maximum phonation times. Therapy goals focused on resonance therapy and vocal volume tasks, such as forward focus "molm" gesture, varying the volume from soft-loud-soft. The final sessions of voice therapy targeted carryover to conversational speech. Audrey demonstrated difficulty using appropriate pitch during connected speech and occasionally returned to her former pattern of a higher pitched, breathy voice.

Treatment Outcomes

By the completion of therapy, Audrey exhibited mild dysphonia characterized by breathiness, roughness, and decreased volume, with only inconsistent high pitch. Both rigid and flexible stroboscopic examinations revealed improved glottic closure. Audrey and her family continued voice therapy tasks using a home program.

Case 5. Patient: Todd (Therapy to Promote Supraglottic Voice Use)

History

Todd was a 17-year-old male who was seen for an initial voice evaluation due to complaints of a chronic "breathy" voice and breathing difficulties during exertion. The patient's medical history was significant for prematurity (25-week premature infant), intubation, tracheostomy for 2 years, and eventually an airway reconstruction surgical procedure with decannulation.

Voice Evaluation

Rigid and flexible stroboscopic examinations revealed that Todd's phonation source was his true vocal folds. A large posterior gap was noted and arytenoid movement was re-

stricted bilaterally. Todd presented with severe dysphonia characterized by breathiness. He subsequently underwent another airway reconstruction procedure, and voice therapy was initiated closer to Todd's home following surgery.

Summary of the Treatment Procedures

Todd's treatment procedure included VFEs, resonance therapy, and phonation tasks emphasizing increased maximum phonation times. He was seen for a voice evaluation 2 months post-initiation of voice therapy and airway reconstruction surgery. Todd continued to present with aphonia and severe dysphonia characterized by breathiness. His voice clinician indicated minimal progress during therapy. Vibratory characteristics were visible only on the anterior portion of the true vocal folds, and a persistent large posterior gap was seen. Although Todd was able to produce short segments of sustained phonation using the true vocal folds, he continued to use a "whispered" confidential voice (aphonia) in connected speech. Following another airway reconstruction surgery, tasks for eliciting supraglottic phonation were attempted during a subsequent voice evaluation. Visible movement of the supraglottic tissue was observed, and at the sustained sound level, the patient's secondary voice was stronger and more functional than his primary voice (true vocal folds). Therapy was continued with Todd's local SLP, who utilized new therapy goals focusing on eliciting and increasing use of his supraglottic voice.

Treatment Outcomes

A follow-up voice evaluation, which occurred 3 months after the second course of voice therapy, revealed a significantly improved perceptual voice. Todd demonstrated consistent progress in the production of his secondary, supraglottic voice. He succeeded across a therapy hierarchy beginning at the single sound level and progressing through the syllable, word, sentence, and connected speech levels. Although Todd was often reluctant to use his secondary voice with peers and across various environments, he continued to demonstrate progress with carryover. Todd and his family agreed that although his secondary voice was rough, with a lower pitch than a "typical" voice, it was functional, whereas his primary voice had not been. Voice therapy continued with goals to further increase the use of Todd's secondary, supraglottic voice.

Case 6. Patient: Zachary (Bilateral Vocal Fold Paralysis)

History

Zachary was a 9-year-old male who had congenital, bilateral vocal fold paralysis. He had a history of several airway surgeries, including a posterior graft and right vocal fold lateralization. He had several courses of voice therapy when he was 5 and 6 years old that resulted in limited improvement. His initial therapy goals focused on decreasing inhalation phonation and initiating the use of an amplification system.

Voice Evaluation

A flexible stroboscopic examination revealed bilateral vocal fold paralysis with an adequate airway. During phonation, incomplete glottic closure and moderate supraglottic compression were revealed. When Zachary was asked to produce a loud voice, he used his supraglottic soft tissues. However, his habitual voice was a whisper. Trial therapy procedures were completed during the evaluation with a successful outcome. Two voices emerged: a low, rough voice and a higher, smoother voice.

Due to these findings, further voice therapy was recommended. Additionally, vocal fold injection was discussed in the event that voice therapy was not completely successful. Voice therapy was recommended for 8 weeks. Zachary was asked to return for a reevaluation in 3 months, or sooner if a plateau in voice therapy was noted.

Summary of the Treatment Procedures

Since Zachary used a whisper as his habitual voice, his initial goal was to consistently use a louder voice in therapy. As he demonstrated the use of two different voices during his evaluation, the voice that was easier to produce was targeted. To help Zachary produce a "voice," he had to "growl" first. Therefore, a growl was used at the beginning of each therapy task for the first few sessions. Once he was comfortable using this voice in therapy, he was asked to begin to generalize his voice use to other environments—first at home and then in conversation with his close friends. This carryover aspect was the most difficult part for Zachary. Therefore, his best friend came to several therapy sessions. The presence of a friend greatly improved the generalization of his louder voice outside of the therapy room. While targeting use of a nonwhisper voice outside of therapy, the clinician also began to work on reducing the roughness of Zachary's voice during sessions by targeting the slightly higher, breathy voice. Forward focus and resonance therapy techniques, such as pitch glides upward with a kazoo, sustaining his higher voice, and humming, were trained. Table 6–1 outlines the progression of exercises performed.

Treatment Outcomes

When Zachary initiated voice therapy, he consistently spoke with a whisper. He completed six 30-minute therapy sessions over

Table 6–1. Progression of Exercises

Exercise	Step 1	Step 2	Step 3
Kazoo	Glide up	Glide up and hold	Produce higher voice without glide
Voice	Growl	Growl and glide up	Produce smoother voice without growl or glide
Hum	Hum+vowel	Hum+words/phrases	Hum+sentences
Generalizing	Use with family members in therapy and at home	Use with close friends in therapy and at home	Begin to use with family members and friends outside of home

a 14-week period, and upon completion he used a low-pitched, rough voice consistently in the therapy room and in comfortable environments. Additionally, he was able to produce a higher, smoother voice more easily when asked to do so in the therapy room. Zachary struggled with generalization, which entailed switching from a whisper to using either of his louder voices in social situations.

Case 7. Patient: Jeff (Subglottic Stenosis and Airway Reconstruction)

History

Jeff was a 7-year-old boy with a long history of subglottic stenosis. He had undergone multiple airway procedures, including a laryngotracheal reconstruction and a cricotracheal resection, but he remained with a tracheostomy. The last airway procedure was a single stage laryngotracheal reconstruction, and he was successfully decannulated. His mother indicated that his classmates were drawn to his rough voice and, unfortunately, often referred to him as a "monster."

Voice Evaluation

Jeff's initial assessment indicated a severe degree of dysphonia marked by severe roughness, low pitch, moderate to severe degree of strain, mild breathiness, and mildly reduced intensity. The stroboscopic examination revealed significant anterior-to-posterior compression of the supraglottic structures, which was the source of voicing. Bilateral arytenoid motion was detected; however, range of motion appeared reduced. The true vocal folds could not be visualized during the examination; however, visualization of the vocal folds in the operating room revealed bilateral, severe scarring. Additionally, Jeff presented with numerous articulation errors, involving glottal stops, velars, fricatives, and plosives.

Summary of the Treatment Procedures

Therapy was initiated by facilitating a forward focus voice with a bilabial lip buzz and voicing while blowing bubbles. Progress was slow, but eventually Jeff was able to produce a less rough, higher pitched voice. Due to the distance he had to travel, voice therapy was transferred to the school-based SLP, with frequent communication between her and the hospital-based SLP. Jeff had success with his new voice in therapy and in the classroom, but he continued to use the lower, rough voice at home. Family counseling revealed that the family had acclimated to the lower pitched voice and their motivation to work on the newer voice was limited. Jeff also identified his lower pitched voice as his "real voice." When this was identified and reasons for making the change were discussed, family involvement improved. He slowly began to use the newer voice more at home. Due to a decrease in the intensity of the new voice, the family petitioned the school and was granted a voice amplifier (ChatterVox).

Treatment Outcomes

Jeff was reassessed several times at the children's hospital voice clinic. His last stroboscopic assessment revealed a severe anterior-to-posterior supraglottic compression that was noted with fixed bilateral arytenoid joints. The vibration source was his arytenoid cartilages against his epiglottis. No other laryngeal functions could be rated. Under simulated, slow motion stroboscopy, mucosal wave was noted on the medial arytenoid tissue for the higher pitched phonation. Lower-pitched phonation was noted using the same arytenoid tissue and the ventricular folds. When Jeff was last seen, he continued to use a supraglottic voice production for both the rougher and smoother voices. However, the hyperfunction of the laryngeal mechanism during production of the smoother voice was noticeably decreased. Jeff used the

two voices interchangeably, reverting to the rougher voice when he needed "power" for his voice.

Chapter Summary

A variety of indirect and direct pediatric voice treatments were presented in this chapter. These treatments were discussed and applied in seven cases presented at the end of the chapter. These cases included vocal fold lesions, bilateral vocal fold paralysis, laryngeal web, subglottic stenosis/airway reconstruction, and functional voice loss. Appendix 6–H contains the DVD's table of content for specific treatment demonstrations with children. Technology relative to computer-based gaming and applications that are used in pediatric voice therapy were identified in this chapter. Telehealth initiatives in pediatric voice treatment were noted, and issues related to the pediatric performing voice were delineated.

References

Abitbol, J., Abitbol, P., & Abitbol, B. (1999). Sex hormones and the female voice. *Journal of Voice, 13*(3), 424–446.

Andrews, M. L. (1997). The singing/acting child: A speech-language pathologist's perspective. *Journal of Voice, 11*(2), 130–134.

Andrews, M. L. (2002). *Voice treatment for children and adolescents.* San Diego, CA: Singular Publishing Group.

Appelman, D. R. (1967). *The science of vocal pedagogy; Theory and application.* Bloomington, IN: Indiana University Press.

Atkinson, D. S. (2010). The effects of choral formation on the singing voice. *Choral Journal, 50*(8), 24–33.

Babad, E. (1993). Pygmalion 25 years after: Interpersonal expectations in the classroom. In P. Blanck (Ed.), *Interpersonal Expectations: Theory, research, and applications* (pp. 125–153). Cambridge, UK: Cambridge University Press.

Barlow, C. A., & Howard, D. M. (2002). Voice source changes of child and adolescent subjects undergoing singing training: A preliminary study. *Logopedics, Phoniatrics & Vocology, 27*(2), 66–73.

Barlow, C., & Howard, D. M. (2005). Electrolaryngographically derived voice source changes of child and adolescent singers. *Logopedics, Phoniatrics & Vocology, 30*(3–4), 147–157.

Becker, M., & Maiman, L. (1975). Sociobehavioral determinants of compliance with health and medical care recommendations. *Medical Care, 13*(1), 10–24.

Behrman, A. (2008). Lip buzzes. In A. Behrman & J. Haskell (Eds.), *Exercises for voice therapy* (pp. 37–38). San Diego, CA: Plural Publishing.

Beijer, L. J., Rietveld, T., Hoskam, V., Geurts, A., & de Swart, B. (2009). Evaluating the feasibility and the potential efficacy of e-learning-based speech therapy (EST) as a Web application for speech training in dysarthric patients with parkinson's disease: A case study. *Telemedicine and e-Health, 16,* 732–738.

Benninger, M. S. (2011). The professional voice. *Journal of Laryngology and Otology, 125*(2), 111–116.

Berry, D. A., Verdolini, K., Montequin, D., Hess, M. M., Chan, R. W., & Titze, I. R. (2001). A quantitative output-cost ratio in voice production. *Journal of Speech, Language, and Hearing Research, 44*(1), 29–37.

Blatt, I. M. (1983). Training singing children during the phases of voice mutation. *Annals of Otology, Rhinology, and Laryngology, 92*(5–1), 462–468.

Boltezar, I. H., Burger, Z. R., & Zargi, M. (1997). Instability of voice in adolescence: pathologic condition or normal developmental variation? *Journal of Pediatrics, 130*(2), 185–190.

Bonet, M., & Casan, P. (1994). Evaluation of dysphonia in a children's choir. *Folia Phoniatrica et Logopaedica, 46*(1), 27–34.

Boseley, M. E., & Hartnick, C. J. (2006). Development of the human true vocal fold: Depth of cell layers and quantifying cell types within the lamina propria. *Annals of Otology, Rhinology and Laryngology, 115*(10), 784–788.

Brown, O. (1996). *Discover your voice: how to develop healthy vocal habits.* San Diego, CA: Singular Publishing Group.

Collins, D. L. (2006). Rehearsal break: Preferred practices in teaching boys whose voices are changing. *Choral Journal, 47*(5), 119–121.

Constintanescu, G. A., Theodoros, D. G., Russell, T. G., Ward, E. C., Wilson, S. J., & Wootton, R. (2011). Treating disordered speech and voice in Parkinson's disease online: A randomized controlled non-inferiority trial. *International Journal of Language and Communication Disorders, 46,* 1–16.

Cooksey, J. M. (1999). *Working with adolescent voices.* St. Louis, MO: Concordia.

Cornut, G., Riou-Bourret, V., & Louis, M. H. (1971). Study of the speaking and singing voice in normal children between 5 and 9 years of age. *Folia Phoniatrica (Basel), 23*(6), 381–389.

Decoster, W., Ghesquiere, S., & Van Steenberge, S. (2008). Great talent, excellent voices—no problem for pubertal girls? *Logopedics, Phoniatrics, & Vocology, 33*(2), 104–112.

Dejonckere, P. H. Wieneke, G. H., Bloemenkamp, D., & LeBacq, J. (1996). F_0-perturbation and F_0/loudness dynamics in voices of normal children, with and without education in singing. *International Journal of Pediatric Otorhinolaryngology, 35*(2), 107–115.

Denizoglu, I., & Sihvo, M. (2010). Lax Vox voice therapy technique. *Current Practice in Otorhinolaryngology, 6,* 285–295.

Echternach, M., Sundberg, J., Arndt, S., Markl, M., Schumacher, M., & Richter, B. (2010). Vocal tract in female registers—a dynamic real-time MRI study. *Journal of Voice, 24,* 133–139.

Edwin, R. (1995). Vocal parenting. *Journal of Singing, 51*(1), 53–56.

Edwin, R. (1997). The singing teacher as vocal parent. *Journal of Voice, 11*(2), 135–137.

Edwin, R. (2001). Vocal exercises for children of all ages. *Journal of Singing, 57*(4), 49–51.

Fatterpekar, G. M., Mukherji, S. K., Rajgopalan, P., Lin, Y., & Castillo, M. (2004). Normal age related signal change in the laryngeal cartilages. *Neuroradiology, 46*(8), 678–681.

Fitch, W. T., & Giedd, J. (1999). Morphology and development of the human vocal tract: A study using magnetic resonance imaging. *Journal of the Acoustical Society of America, 106*(3), 1511–1522.

Friar, K. K. (1999). Changing voices, changing times. *Music Educators Journal, 86*(3), 26–29.

Gartner-Schmidt, J. L. (2010). Flow phonation. In J. Stemple & L. Fry (Eds.), *Voice therapy: Clinical studies* (3rd ed., pp. 84–92). San Diego, CA: Plural Publishing.

Gauffin J., & Sundberg, J. (1989). Spectral correlates of glottal voice source waveform characteristics. *Journal of Speech, Language, and Hearing Research, 32*, 556–565.

Good, T. (1987). Two decades of research on teacher expectations: Findings and future directions. *Journal of Teacher Education, 38*(4), 32–47.

Grogan-Johnson, S., Alvares, R., Rowan, L., & Creaghead, N. (2010). A pilot study comparing the effectiveness of speech language therapy provided by telemedicine with conventional on-site therapy. *Journal of Telemedicine and Telecare, 16*, 134–139.

Hartnick, C., & Boseley, M. (2008). *Pediatric voice disorders: Diagnosis and treatment.* San Diego, CA: Plural Publishing.

Hartnick, C. J., Rehbar, R., & Prasad, V. (2005). Development and maturation of the pediatric human vocal fold lamina propria. *Laryngoscope, 115*(1), 4–15.

Hasek, C. S., Singh, S., & Murry, T. (1980). Acoustic attributes of preadolescent voices. *Journal of the Acoustical Society of America, 68*(5), 1262–1265.

Hollien, H. (2011). On pubescent voice change in males. *Journal of Voice, 26*(2), 1–12.

Hook, S. (1998). Changing voice and middle school music: An interview with John Cooksey and Nancy Cox. *Choral Journal, 39*(1), 21–26.

Kahane, J. C. (1978). A morphological study of the human prepubertal and pubertal larynx. *American Journal of Anatomy, 151*(1), 11–19.

Kahane, J., & Mayo, R. (1989). The need for aggressive pursuit of healthy childhood voices. *Language, Speech, and Hearing Services in Schools, 20*, 102–107.

KayPENTAX Instruction Manual Issue F. (2009). Visi-Pitch IV, Model 3950B & Sona-Speech II, Model 3650. KayPENTAX, Montvale, NJ.

Killian, J. (1999). A description of vocal maturation among fifth- and sixth-grade boys. *Journal of Research in Music Education, 47*(4), 357–369.

King, S. N., Davis, L., Lehman, J. L., & Ruddy, B. H. (2012). A model for treating voice disorders in school-age children within a video gaming environment. *Journal of Voice, 26*(5), 656–663.

Kotby, M. N., Shiromoto, O., & Hirano, M. (1993). The accent method of voice therapy: Effect of accentuations on F_0, SPL, and airflow. *Journal of Voice, 7*(4), 319–325.

Lee, L., Pennington, E., & Stemple, J. (1998). Leading roles in a high school musical: Effects on objective and subjective measures of vocal production. *Medical Problems of Performing Artists, 13*(4), 167–171.

Lessac, A. (1997). *The use and training of the human voice: A biodynamic approach to vocal life.* Mountain View, CA: Mayfield Publishing.

Lundy, D., Roy, S., Casiano, R., Xue, J., & Evans, J. (2000). Acoustic analysis of the singing and speaking voice in singing students. *Journal of Voice, 14*(4), 490–493.

Maira, C., Hapner, E., & Olson, B. (2012, June). "There's an app for that." Workshop conducted at the Voice Foundation Symposium, Philadelphia, PA.

McAllister, A., Sederholm, E., Sundberg, J., & Gramming, P. (1994). Relations between voice range profiles and physiological and perceptual voice characteristics in ten-year-old children. *Journal of Voice, 8*(3), 230–239.

McAllister, A., & Sundberg, J. (1998). Data on subglottal pressure and SPL at varied vocal loudness and pitch in 8- to 11-year-old children. *Journal of Voice, 12*(2), 166–174.

McKenzie, D. (1956). The boy's changing voice. *Music Journal, 14*(9), 29–39.

McNamara, A. P., & Perry, C. K. (1994). Vocal abuse prevention practices: A national survey of school-based speech-language pathologists. *Language, Speech, and Hearing Services in Schools, 25,* 105–111.

Mecke, A. C., & Sundberg, J. (2010). Gender differences in children's singing voices: Acoustic analyses and results of a listening test. *Journal of the Acoustical Society of America, 127*(5), 3223–3231.

Miller, R. (1995). Breathy young female voices. *Journal of Singing, 51*(5), 37–39.

Miller, R. (1996). *The structure of singing: System and art in vocal technique.* New York, NY: Schirmer Books.

Miller, R. (2000). *Training soprano voices.* New York, NY: Oxford University Press.

Miller, R. (2009). Voice pedagogy: in the beginning: The genesis of the art of singing. *Journal of Singing—the Official Journal of the National Association of Teachers of Singing, 66*(1), 45–50.

Møller, K. (2006). The Accent Method. Retrieved from http://www.voicesource.co.uk /article/180.

Nienkerke-Springer, A., McAllister, A., & Sundberg. J. (2005). Effects of family therapy on children's voices. *Journal of Voice, 19*(1), 103–113.

Overby, M., Carrell, T., & Bernthal, J. (2007). Teachers' perceptions of students with speech sound disorders: A quantitative and qualitative analysis. *American Speech-Language-Hearing Association, 38,* 327–341.

Pedersen, M., Møller, S., Krabbe, S., Munk, E., & Bennett, P. (1985). A multivariate statistical analysis of voice phenomena related to puberty in choir boys. *Folia Phoniatrica, 37,* 271–278.

Phillips, K. H. (1992). *Teaching kids to sing.* New York, NY: Schirmer Books.

Reilly, J. S. (1995). The three ages of voice: The "singing-acting" child: The laryngologist's perspective, 1995. *Journal of Voice, 11*(2), 126–129.

Ripich, D. (1989). Building classroom communication competence: A case for a multiperspective approach. *Seminars in Speech and Language, 10,* 231–240.

Roy, N., Gray, S., Simon, M., Dove, H., Corbin-Lewis, K., & Stemple, J. (2001). An evaluation of the effects of two treatment approaches for teachers with voice disorders: A prospective randomized clinical trial. *Journal of Speech, Language, and Hearing Research, 44*(2), 286–296.

Roy, N., Weinrich, B., Gray, S., Tanner, K., Stemple, J., & Sapienza, C. (2003). Three treatments for teachers with voice disorders: A randomized clinical trial. *Journal of Speech, Language, and Hearing Research, 46*(3), 670–688.

Ruddy, B. H., & Sapienza, C. M. (2004). Treating voice disorders in a school-based setting: Working within the framework of IDEA. *Language, Speech, and Hearing Services in Schools, 35*(4), 327–332.

Rutkowski, J., & Miller, M. S. (2002). A longitudinal study of elementary children's acquisition of their singing voices. *Update: Applications of Research in Music Education, 22*(1), 5–14.

Sabol, J., Lee, L., & Stemple, J. (1995). Efficacy of vocal function exercises in the practice regimen of singers. *Journal of Voice, 9*(1), 27–36.

Sataloff, R. (1998). *Vocal health and pedagogy.* San Diego, CA: Singular Publishing Group.

Schneider, B., Zumtobel, M., Prettenhofer, W., Aichstill, B., & Jocher, W. (2010). Normative voice range profiles in vocally trained and untrained children aged between 7 and 10 years. *Journal of Voice, 24*(2), 153–160.

Sergeant, D. C., & Welch, G. F. (2009). Gender differences in long-term average spectra of children's singing voices. *Journal of Voice, 23*(3), 319–336.

Siupsinskiene, N., & Lycke, H. (2011). Effects of vocal training on singing and speaking voice characteristics in vocally healthy adults and children based on choral and nonchoral data. *Journal of Voice, 25*(4), 177–189.

Skadsem, J. A. (2007). Singing through the voice change. *General Music Today, 21*(1), 32–34.

Skelton, K. D. (2007). The child's voice: A closer look at pedagogy and science. *Journal of Singing, 63*(5), 537–544.

Spremulli, M. (2008). Voice Aerobics™. Retrieved from http://www.voiceaerobicsdvd.com/.

Stemple, J., Glaze, L., & Klaben, B. (2010). *Clinical voice pathology: Theory and management* (4th ed.). San Diego, CA: Plural Publishing.

Stemple, J., Lee, L., D'Amico, B., & Pickup, B. (1994). Efficacy of vocal function exercises as a method of improving voice production. *Journal of Voice, 8*(3), 271–278.

Stone, R. E., & Casteel, R. L. (1982). Intervention in non-organically based dysphonia. In M. Filter (Ed.), *Phonatory disorders in children* (pp. 166–180). New York, NY: CC Thomas.

Swanson, F. (1984). Changing voices: Don't leave out the boys. *Music Educators Journal, 70*(5), 47–50.

Tepe, E. S., Deutsch, E. S., Sampson, Q., Lawless, S., Reilly, J. S., & Sataloff, R. T. (2002). A pilot survey of vocal health in young singers. *Journal of Voice, 16*(2), 244–250.

Titze, I. R. (2006). Voice training and therapy with a semi-occluded vocal tract: Rationale and scientific underpinnings. *Journal of Speech, Language, and Hearing Research, 49,* 448–459.

Trollinger, V. (2007). Pediatric vocal development and voice science: Implications for teaching singing. *General Music Today, 20*(3), 19–25.

Vennard, W. (1967). *Singing, the mechanism and technique.* New York, NY: Carl Fischer.

Verdolini Abbott, K. (1998). *Resonant voice therapy.* Iowa City, IA: National Center for Voice and Speech.

Verdolini Abbott, K. (2012a). *A voice therapy spectrum* [Pamphlet]. Kankakee, IL: Multi Voice Dimensions.

Verdolini Abbott, K. (2012b). *Adventures in voice. A workshop for speech-language pathologists* [Pamphlet]. Kankakee, IL: Multi Voice Dimensions.

Verduyckt, I., Remacle, M., Jamart, J., Benderitter, C., & Morsomme, D. (2011). Voice-related complaints in the pediatric population. *Journal of Voice, 25(3)*, 373–380.

Weinrich, B. (2002). Common voice disorders in children. *Perspectives on Voice and Voice Disorders, 12*(1), 13–16.

Welch, G. (1988). Beginning singing with young children. *Journal of Singing, 45,* 12–15.

Whiteside, S. P., Hodgson, C., & Tapster, C. (2002). Vocal characteristics in preadolescent and adolescent children: A longitudinal study. *Logopedics, Phoniatrics & Vocology, 27*(1), 12–20.

Williams, B., Larson, G., & Price, D. (1996). An investigation of selected female singing- and speaking-voice characteristics through a comparison of pre-menarcheal girls to a group of post-menarcheal girls. *Journal of Singing, 52*(1), 33–40.

Williams, J., Welch, G., & Howard, D. (2005). An exploratory baseline study of boy chorister vocal behaviour and development in an intensive professional context. *Logopedic, Phoniatric & Vocology, 20,* 158–162.

Yarnell, S. (2006). Vocal and aural perceptions of young singers aged ten to twenty-one. *Journal of Singing, 63*(1), 81–85.

Zacharias, S. R. C., Kelchner, L., & Creaghead, N. (2013). Teachers' perceptions of adolescent females with voice disorders. *Language, Speech, and Hearing Services in Schools, 44*(2), 174–182.

APPENDIX 6–A

Vocal Hygiene Guidelines

Certain behaviors are harmful to the vocal folds, which may play a part in your child's voice disorder. You and your child should recognize these vocally abusive behaviors and modify, reduce, or stop them. This will help to heal the vocal folds and produce the best results for improved voice.

You can help your child modify, reduce, or stop the following vocally abusive behaviors	*Possible solutions:*
Using a loud voice or yelling to get someone's attention. For example, the child attempts to talk to a family member who is upstairs while the child is downstairs.	Have your child walk to the person, wave, or tap on his or her shoulder Then talk to the person in a gentle, softer voice instead of yelling. Text person with phone
Yelling and screaming during play activities, such as during recess, gym class, or sports events	Use a gentle, softer voice instead of yelling. If louder voice is needed, have good breath support from your belly and use a comfortable, lower pitch.
Talking at the same time as others (This results in increased volume.)	Take turns talking with your child. Do not interrupt or talk at the same time.
Whispering instead of talking	Use a gentle, soft voice (as used in a library) instead of a whisper voice (i.e., child version of confidential voice).
Using a voice that is too high or too low	Use a medium, comfortable pitch. Let voice glide down to a comfortable pitch if it is too high (and glide up if too low).

continued

You can help your child modify, reduce, or stop the following vocally abusive behaviors	Possible solutions:
Frequent coughing or throat clearing	Swallow long and hard 2 or 3 times (with or without liquid) or use gentle, nonvoiced throat clearing. Also increase water intake
Using a squeaky, strained vocal quality	Practice neck rolls or drop and relax the jaw. Try to relax throat muscles when humming. Use a medium, lower pitched voice.
Using loud, abusive play sounds (for example, animal or motor sounds)	Use words when playing instead of abusive sounds. Use different sounds, such as raspberries or whistle.
Additional guidelines:	
Drink at least 5 cups of water each day	Stay out of smoky places.
Avoid caffeine (found in colas, other sodas/pops, coffee, tea, chocolate)	

Source: Modified and used courtesy of Cincinnati Children's Hospital Medical Center, Division of Speech-Language Pathology.

APPENDIX 6–B

Vocal Hygiene Record

Please circle or enter response (in the appropriate box) for the following behaviors:

	Date:	*Date:*	*Date:*	*Date:*	*Date:*	*Date:*	*Date:*
Throat clearing	y/n	y/n	y/n	y/n	y/n	y/n	y/n
Speaking loudly	y/n	y/n	y/n	y/n	y/n	y/n	y/n
Yelling/ screaming	y/n	y/n	y/n	y/n	y/n	y/n	y/n
Speaking for a prolonged period of time	y/n	y/n	y/n	y/n	y/n	y/n	y/n
Glottal fry	y/n	y/n	y/n	y/n	y/n	y/n	y/n
Hard glottal attacks	y/n	y/n	y/n	y/n	y/n	y/n	y/n
Water intake	___cups	___cups	___cups	___cups	___cups	___cups	___cups
Caffeine intake	___cups	___cups	___cups	___cups	___cups	___cups	___cups
Smoking/smoky environments	y/n	y/n	y/n	y/n	y/n	y/n	y/n

Source: Modified and used courtesy of Cincinnati Children's Hospital Medical Center, Division of Speech-Language Pathology.

Gastroesophageal Reflux Information for Families

What is gastroesophageal reflux?

Gastroesophageal reflux occurs when stomach contents reflux, or return, into the esophagus (the tube that connects the throat to the stomach), during or after a meal. In some children, the stomach contents go up into the mouth and are swallowed again. This may result in hoarseness, recurrent pneumonia, chronic cough, wheezing, and trouble breathing or swallowing.

What causes reflux?

There is a ring of muscle at the bottom of the esophagus that opens and closes. It allows food to enter the stomach. When this muscle opens, stomach contents and acid can enter into the esophagus, causing reflux. When reflux occurs often or does not clear from the esophagus, the lining of the esophagus can become damaged.

How does reflux affect the voice?

Sometimes acid reflux spills over into the larynx (voice box). Acid reflux into the larynx and throat is often called laryngopharyngeal reflux, or LPR. Acid that reaches the larynx can irritate the vocal folds. This causes them to swell. This also disrupts their normal vibration. Even small amounts of acid can cause damage. Symptoms of LPR include hoarseness, a "lump in the throat," throat pain, postnasal drip, frequent throat clearing, excessive throat mucus, a sore throat, and/or a cough.

How is reflux treated?

Treatment varies depending on the child's symptoms and age. Medication may help to decrease the amount of acid made in the stomach. Dietary and lifestyle changes may also help to reduce symptoms.

Home suggestions for dietary/ lifestyle changes

- Provide small but frequent meals all day.
- Avoid overeating.
- Avoid foods that can aggravate reflux.
- Avoid tight-fitting clothing, especially around the stomach.
- Limit high level physical activity for at least one hour after eating.
- Keep your child upright for at least half an hour after eating.
- Feed your child at least 2 hours before bedtime or naptime.
- Raise the head of the bed from the floor level. This helps to keep stomach contents from traveling to the larynx.

Foods that can aggravate reflux

- Vegetables (due to high acid or belching): broccoli, green peppers, cabbage, brussel sprouts, cauliflower, corn, cucumber, onion, and garlic

- Fruits (due to high acid or lots of fiber and seeds): tomatoes and tomato-based products (pasta sauce or pizza), apples (especially peels), citrus fruits, figs, bananas, and coconuts
- Beverages: carbonated and/or caffeinated drinks, citrus juices (orange juice, grapefruit juice, etc.) hot chocolate, milk (if lactose intolerant), coffee (even decaffeinated), and tea
- Starches: beans (gas producing), oats (exception: rolled oats), and tofu in large quantities
- Miscellaneous: fatty or fried foods; meat with connective tissue/gristle; chili powder and other spicy foods; vinegars; chocolates; molasses; peppermint/spearmint; cough drops; honey; foods with "air," such as fluffy baked goods (meringues); rye seeds; meat extracts; black pepper (exception: white pepper); creamy foods (high fat content); and pastries (high fat content).

Modified and used courtesy of Cincinnati Children's Hospital Medical Center, Division of Speech-Language Pathology.

APPENDIX 6–D

Vocal Function Exercises Home Instructions

Voice production requires three activities:

- Breath support
- Phonation (vibration of vocal cords)
- Resonance (sound vibrations in the throat, mouth, and nose)

Children with a voice disorder often develop an imbalance of these three systems. An imbalance can result in a rough, strained voice quality. The goal of Vocal Function Exercises is to balance all three parts of the vocal mechanism. Your child's speech-language pathologist will work with you and your child on these exercises. It is important to practice these exercises only under the direction of a speech-language pathologist.

Have the child complete each of the following exercises two times each and two times per day, once in the morning and once in the evening. Begin each exercise with a deep breath through the nose.

- Sustain "eeee" for as long as possible on the musical note _____. The sound should be produced through the nose. This is a warm-up activity. **GOAL:** _____ seconds.

(Record the sustained time on your data sheet for each time this exercise is done.)

- Glide from your lowest note to your highest note using the word "whoop." The sound should vibrate the lips. This should be similar to the sound of a kazoo and should make the lips tingle. If this is difficult to produce, try producing a "raspberry" sound with the lips vibrating and glide from low sounds to high sounds. This stretches the "voice" muscles. **GOAL:** No pitch breaks.

- Glide from your highest note to your lowest note using the word "boom." Again, the sound should vibrate the lips. This contracts the "voice" muscles. **GOAL:** No pitch breaks.

- Sustain the musical notes ___, ___, ___, ___, ___ for as long as possible saying "ol." This should be similar to the sound of a kazoo and should make the lips tingle. It is important to keep the lips rounded. Do each note as softly as possible. This is a power building activity. **GOAL:** _____ seconds. (Record the sustained time on your data sheet for each time this exercise is done.)

Modified and used courtesy of Cincinnati Children's Hospital Medical Center, Division of Speech-Language Pathology.

Vocal Function Exercises Data Form

Begin with deep breath through the nose. Produce note as softly as possible. Record # of seconds [s] each note was sustained.

For glides, circle "+" to indicate no pitch break; circle "–" to indicate pitch break occurred.

	Date:		Date:		Date:		Date:		Date:	
	A.M.	*P.M.*	*A.M.*	*P.M.*	*A.M.*	*P.M.*	*A.M.*	*P.M.*	*A.M.*	*P.M.*
Match note___ Nasal vowel "ee"	____s	____s	____s	____s	____s	____s	____s	____s	____s	____s
	____s	____s	____s	____s	____s	____s	____s	____s	____s	____s
*Glide up "whoop" or lip vibration	+ / –	+ / –	+ / –	+ / –	+ / –	+ / –	+ / –	+ / –	+ / –	+ / –
	+ / –	+ / –	+ / –	+ / –	+ / –	+ / –	+ / –	+ / –	+ / –	+ / –
Glide down "boom" or lip vibration	+ / –	+ / –	+ / –	+ / –	+ / –	+ / –	+ / –	+ / –	+ / –	+ / –
	+ / –	+ / –	+ / –	+ / –	+ / –	+ / –	+ / –	+ / –	+ / –	+ / –
Match note ___ "ol" lips rounded	____s	____s	____s	____s	____s	____s	____s	____s	____s	____s
	____s	____s	____s	____s	____s	____s	____s	____s	____s	____s
Match note ___ "ol" lips rounded	____s	____s	____s	____s	____s	____s	____s	____s	____s	____s
	____s	____s	____s	____s	____s	____s	____s	____s	____s	____s

continued

	Date:		Date:		Date:		Date:		Date:	
	A.M.	P.M.	A.M.	P.M.	A.M.	P.M.	A.M.	P.M.	A.M.	P.M.
Match note ___ "ol" lips rounded	___s	___s	___s	___s	___s	___s	___s	___s	___s	___s
	___s	___s	___s	___s	___s	___s	___s	___s	___s	___s
Match note ___ "ol" lips rounded	___s	___s	___s	___s	___s	___s	___s	___s	___s	___s
	___s	___s	___s	___s	___s	___s	___s	___s	___s	___s
Match note ___ "ol" lips rounded	___s	___s	___s	___s	___s	___s	___s	___s	___s	___s
	___s	___s	___s	___s	___s	___s	___s	___s	___s	___s

Source: Modified and used courtesy of Cincinnati Children's Hospital Medical Center, Division of Speech-Language Pathology.

APPENDIX 6–F

Resonance Therapy Home Instructions

Note: Begin each exercise with a deep breath through the nose.

Step #1

- Say "holm-molm-molm-molm-molm-molm" as a sigh, from a higher to lower pitch and ending with a comfortable pitch
  - Exercise should be comfortable and relaxing
  - Be sure to use a lot of breath to support the sound
  - Focus on the narrow vibration, "like a narrow beam of light"

Step #2

- Say "molm-molm-molm" with a comfortable pitch
  - Vary the rate (slow-fast-slow)
  - Vary the intensity (soft-loud-soft)

Step #3

- Say "molm-molm-molm" as speech

- Say these words in the same way as you would a sentence
- Vary the rate, pitch, and loudness as if you're speaking to someone

Step #4

- Chant the following sentences with a comfortable pitch:
  - Mary made me mad.
  - My mother made marmalade.
  - My mom may marry Marv.
  - My merry mom may marry Marv.
  - Marv made my mother merry.
- Say each sentence with extra inflection
- Say each sentence in a natural speech-like manner

Step #5

- Say "mamapapa-mamapapa" with a comfortable pitch
  - Vary the rate (slow-fast-slow)
  - Vary the intensity (soft-loud-soft)
  - Vary rate, pitch, loudness as if you're speaking to someone

Step #6

- Chant the following sentences with a comfortable pitch:
    - Mom may put Paul on the moon.
    - Mom told Tom to copy my manner.
    - My manner made Pete and Paul mad.
    - Mom may move Polly's movie to ten.
    - My movie made Tim and Tom sad.
- Say each sentence with extra inflection
- Say each sentence in a natural speech-like manner

Step #7

- Say the following sentences with a forward-focus tone of voice:
    - All the girls were laughing.
    - Get there before they close.
    - Did you hear what she said?
    - Come in and close the door.
    - Are you going tonight?
    - Put everything away.
    - Come whenever you can.
    - We heard that yesterday.
    - The player broke his leg.
    - The children went swimming.
- If the forward-focus tone cannot be maintained, use chanting and extra inflection

Step #8

- Practice forward-focus speech with structured and unstructured materials
    - (reading to conversation)

Modified and used courtesy of Cincinnati Children's Hospital Medical Center, Division of Speech-Language Pathology.

APPENDIX 6–G

Resonance Therapy Data Form

Place a check mark (in the appropriate box) when you have completed your 8 to 10-minute home-practice sessions twice per day (i.e., Step 1, Step 2, Step 3). Bring this data sheet to each therapy session.

	Date_____		Date_____		Date_____		Date_____		Date_____		Date_____		Date_____	
Step 1														
Step 2														
Step 3														
Step 4														
Step 5														
Step 6														
Step 7														
Step 8														

Source: Modified and used courtesy of Cincinnati Children's Hospital Medical Center, Division of Speech-Language Pathology.

DVD Table of Contents: Demonstration of Treatment Methods

Vocal Function Exercises Step 1
Vocal Function Exercises Step 2
Vocal Function Exercises Step 3
Vocal Function Exercises Step 4
Vocal Function Exercises With Child Adaptations
    for Front Focus and Pitch Match
Resonance Therapy Steps 1 through 3
Resonance Therapy Steps 4 through 7
Resonance Therapy Step 8
Flow Phonation: Gargling
Flow Phonation: Cup Bubble Blowing &
    Straw Phonation
Flow Phonation: /u/ Prolongation
Lip Buzzes
Healthy Shouting
Accent Method
Example of Telehealth Session

CHAPTER 7

Managing Children with Complex Voice Disorders

Overview

This chapter provides information related to the management and care of children with complex voice disorders secondary to airway injury, structural abnormalities, diseases, and hyperreactivity of the laryngeal airway. Included in this group are children who have undergone tracheotomy with long-term tracheostomy tube placement and subsequent airway reconstruction, children who have had a laryngectomy, and children with the diagnosis of paradoxical vocal fold dysfunction. Although not necessarily considered complex in terms of underlying anatomic changes, puberphonia and childhood muscle tension dysphonia (MTD) as potentially complex functional disorders are included in this chapter.

Pediatric Airway Injury

Modern neonatal medicine has advanced the care and survival rates of premature or similarly medically fragile infants. In the last 30 years the number of preterm births has increased by 30%, resulting in over 500,000 children born before 37 weeks gestation annually (Centers for Disease Control, 2013; March of Dimes, 2013). Despite advances in the respiratory care of premature infants, babies born at or before 28 weeks gestation remain at the greatest risk for respiratory distress syndrome (RDS) and bronchopulmonary dysplasia (BPD) and may require some period of prolonged endotracheal intubation and ventilator support (American Lung Association, 2013). According to the American Lung Association Disease Data from 2008, each year there are approximately 12,000 babies born weighing less than 3.3 pounds who develop BPD.

Endotracheal intubation means that the breathing tube is inserted through the mouth, pharynx, and larynx down into the tracheal airway. Long-term endotracheal intubation can lead to mucosal injury and other oral, pharyngeal, and laryngeal injuries. The reported incidence of diagnosed acquired laryngeal injury in this population during initial hospitalization is varied and may not be detected until after hospital discharge (Carron, Derkay, Strope, Nosonchuk, & Darrow, 2000; Cordeiro, Fernandes, & Troster, 2004; da Silva & Stevens, 1999; Downing & Kilbride, 1995; Lee et al., 2002; Pereira, MacGregor, McDuffie, & Mitchell, 2003; Walner, Loewen, & Kimura, 2001). For infants who require prolonged endotracheal intubation, the decision to have them undergo a tracheotomy is dictated by multiple medical factors, including concomitant health issues and the anticipated length and type of ventilation support needed. In premature or similarly medically fragile infants and children, traumatic or prolonged intubation can result in injury and narrowing of the laryngotracheal airway.

Subglottic Stenosis

Narrowing of the airway is broadly referred to as laryngotracheal stenosis (LTS) or if below the vocal folds, subglottic stenosis (SGS) (Myer, Cotton, & Shott, 1995). SGS can be either acquired or congenital. The degree of narrowing or severity is described according to a grading scale: Grade 1 is classified as a 0 to 50% narrowing of the subglottic area, grade 2 is a 51 to 75% narrowing, grade 3 is a 76 to 99% narrowing, and grade 4 is complete obstruction of the subglottic area (Figure 7–1)(Myer, O'Connor, & Cotton, 1994).

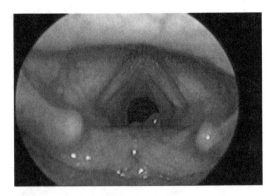

Figure 7–2. Endoscopic view of subglottic stenosis. Image used with permission from the Center for Pediatric Voice Disorders, Cincinnati Children's Hospital, Cincinnati, Ohio.

Congenital SGS is due to some type of embryologic anomaly where there is a failure of the glottic and subglottic region to properly separate. A common cause of acquired SGS is airway injury secondary to prolonged intubation (Figure 7–2).

Pediatric Tracheotomy and Tracheostomy

The terms *tracheotomy* and *tracheostomy* are often interchanged but do have two distinct meanings. *Tracheotomy* refers to the surgical procedure of creating an opening into the tracheal airway at the level of the third or fourth tracheal rings, and *tracheostomy* refers to inserting a tube (cannula) to secure the opening. A tracheotomy provides an alternate airway routing the flow of air for ventilator and respiratory purposes from the upper airway (mouth and nose) to the neck. Placement of a tracheostomy tube keeps the opening (stoma) to the tracheal airway open. Most children who need tracheostomies are less than 1 year of age (Mitchell et al., 2012). In the instance of the very premature infant,

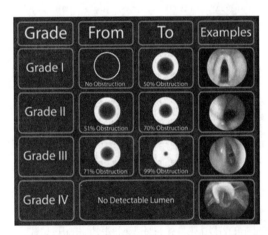

Figure 7–1. Cotton-Myer Grading Scale for Subglottic Stenosis. From *The Pediatric Airway. An Interdisciplinary Approach*, by C. M. Myer III, R. T. Cotton, and S. R. Schott, 1995. Reprinted with permission from Lippincott, Williams & Wilkins.

respiratory distress can necessitate ventilator support for days, weeks, months, or longer. Similarly, in any infant or child, airway emergencies resulting from airway obstruction, acute trauma, severe cardiopulmonary distress, or neurologic insult can require medical surgical management that includes placement of a tracheostomy tube.

Tracheostomy Tubes

There are numerous styles and types of pediatric tracheostomy tubes. A basic pediatric tracheostomy tube has the following component parts: outer cannula, inner cannula, collar or flanges, hub, and obturator (Table 7–1 and Figure 7–3). Optional features can include a cuff and fenestration. If the tracheostomy tube has a cuff, there will also be a pilot line and balloon. Water (saline) or air is infused to fill the cuff. Disposable pediatric tracheostomy tubes are made of silicone and range in sizes that are measured by the size of the inner diameter (ID) and outer diameter (OD) of the cannula (e.g., ID: 2.5–4.0 mm and OD: 4.0–6.0 mm) and length (e.g., 30–36 mm).

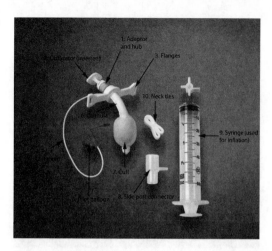

Figure 7–3. Standard component parts of a tracheostomy tube. Image courtesy of Bryan Medical. Used with permission.

See Figure 7–4 for representative samples. On neonatal and infant trach tubes, the tracheostomy tube flange may be straight or V shaped, cuffed (including tight to shaft) or cuffless. Commonly used brands include Bivona®, Shiley®, Portex®, and TRACOE®.

The purpose of the cuff is to seal the lower airway in order to create and maintain

Table 7–1. The Tracheostomy Tube: Parts and Function

Part	Function
Inner cannula	Is inserted into the outer cannula; has the hub; is removable for cleaning
Outer cannula	Is the main structure of the trach tube; functions as the alternate airway; inserted into the trachea; is changed periodically
Flange	Outer collar of the trach tube; has slits for ties
Hub	Outer portion of the trach tube; twists to unlock or lock the inner cannula in place; is the point of attachment for speaking valves
Cuff	Seals the lower airway during ventilation; does not prevent aspiration
Pilot balloon and line	Is used for inflation and deflation of the cuff. A full balloon indicates an inflated cuff and a flat balloon indicates a deflated cuff
Fenestration	Openings in the outer cannula that permit air to flow up through the laryngeal and upper airway upon trach occlusion
"Nosey"/filter	Filters, warms, and humidifies inhaled air

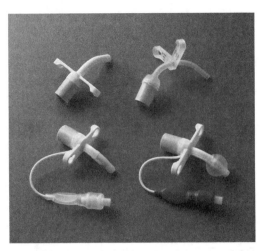

Figure 7–4. Bivona Neonatal pediatric tracheostomy tubes. Note that the lower right trach tube depicts an inflated cuff. Image provided by Smiths-Medical. Used with permission.

the needed pulmonary pressures to inflate the lungs during mechanical ventilation. A cuff may also provide some cushioning of the outer cannula against the tracheal wall. However, overinflation of a cuff can cause tracheal injury. When the cuff is inflated and the seal complete, no air should be able to be directed to and through the upper airway. Of note, some brands of pediatric tracheostomy tubes do not have cuffs.

A fenestrated tube is where there are openings in the outer cannula to permit air to flow up through the larynx and upper airway. The fenestration works only if there are corresponding holes in the inner cannula or the inner cannula is removed. There are concerns about tracheal trauma and granulation formation with fenestrated trach tubes, as the edges of the fenestration can irritate the tracheal wall.

Although the tracheostomy tube may be initially secured by sutures end eventually by ties, it will move within the trachea during movement of the child and ongoing natural bodily functions like swallowing. Excessive movement of the tube can also cause irritation and inflammation of the tracheal wall. Any area of inflammation may lead to tissue injury and scarring, granuloma formation, and development of subglottic stenosis (Figure 7–5). While the child is an inpatient, care and cleaning of the tracheostomy tube is the responsibility of the patient's medical team, although the informed SLP will know the process and procedures. Parents and caregivers typically assume this care when the child is discharged home, although home health support is often needed. Having two individuals present who are trained to provide ongoing and emergency care is recommended.

The Role of the SLP in Caring for the Child With a Tracheostomy

The functional changes created by breathing through a tracheostomy include reduced natural filtering of inhaled air, changes in sensory input to the nose and mouth, potential alteration of pressures in the oropharynx and larynx during swallowing, tracheal injury, and loss of voicing. In an infant, a loss of the ability to vocalize can impact development of overall communication abilities (Jiang & Morrison, 2003; Simon, Fowler, & Handler, 1983). Normal speech and language development is enhanced when the child vocalizes and repeats words; thus the importance of vocal play in the development of speech sounds and the resulting interaction with caretakers is essential for early communication exchange. Loss or restriction of these experiences needs to be addressed through supplemental types of communication experiences such as signing, mouthing words, alternative communication, alternative sound generation, developmental language intervention, and when appropriate, introducing the use of a speaking valve. Providing guidance and intervention for overall communication development is a central function of the SLP on the team (Wood-north, 2004).

> Clinical Note: It is not uncommon for parents or caregivers to attribute a lack of language development to the fact that the child has a tracheostomy tube and cannot voice. If the need for a tracheostomy tube occurs in conjunction with other significant medical and developmental concerns, informing and supporting parents and caregivers about the role that voicing plays in overall communication and language development is essential.

Tracheostomy and Dysphagia

Having a tracheostomy is a known risk factor for dysphagia in young children (Normal, Louw, & Kritzinger, 2007). One of the advantages of a tracheostomy tube is the access to the lower airway for pulmonary toileting (i.e., keeping the lungs clear of excessive secretions via cough and suctioning), and in cases of severe and chronic aspiration, this is absolutely necessary. However, the presence of a tracheostomy tube can also create or contribute to mechanical swallowing and airway protection difficulties. The presence of the tracheal opening for the tracheostomy tube can change the normal pharyngeal pressure events during swallowing. If there are anchoring effects of the tracheostomy tube on the skin and extrinsic strap muscles, the hyoid and larynx may not fully elevate during the swallow. Elevation of the hyolaryngeal complex is an important component of airway protection. If the tracheostomy tube impinges on the esophagus, it can create an obstacle to bolus flow through the esophagus.

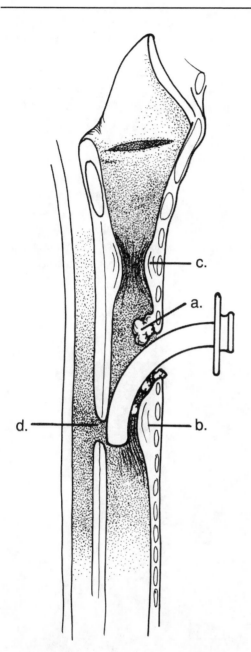

Figure 7–5. Acquired tracheal stenosis may result from granulation tissue (A), cuff pressure (B), improper (high) tracheotomy (C), or in association with posterior tracheal wall necrosis (D). From *The Pediatric Airway. An Interdisciplinary Approach*, by C. M. Myer III, R. T. Cotton, and S. R. Schott, 1995. Reprinted with permission from Lippincott, Williams & Wilkins.

The lack of airflow through the larynx may also diminish airway sensitivity and reactivity (Dikeman & Kazandjian, 2003; Elpern, Borkgren Okonek, Bacon, Gertrung, & Skryzynski, 2000). Lastly, whether the presence of a tracheostomy tube exacerbates any gastroesophageal reflux disease or laryngopharyngeal reflux (LPR) that the child is experiencing warrants consideration and should be ruled out or managed (Normal et al.). Of note, inflating the cuff on a tracheostomy tube does not prevent aspiration but can delay the entry of aspirated oral pharyngeal secretions or prandial material deep into the lungs.

Adult patients can communicate specific discomfort and sensory changes associated with a tracheostomy and its care. In contrast, children may communicate discomfort via behavioral changes such as demonstrating new and negative behaviors associated with feeding, including oral hypersensitivity and food refusal. Discerning whether swallowing problems are secondary to the presence of a tracheostomy tube alone, the need to have a tracheostomy, and/or other health and developmental concerns requires careful examination and excellent diagnostic skills.

Tracheostomy and Voicing

Work on voicing with a tracheostomy tube in place can begin when the child is medically stable and the clinician has received physician authorization. Of primary concern is the child's ability to comfortably exhale air through the upper airway with an occluded trach tube. This requires that the child have an unobstructed laryngeal and upper airway (no lesions, edema, etc.). Directing pulmonary air up through the larynx in order to initiate and sustain vocal fold vibration requires that the child be able to tolerate short periods of trach tube occlusion (with a clean, gloved finger) and have sufficient air leak around the exterior of the outer cannula that can be redirected through the larynx and upper airway (Woodnorth, 2004). If there is a cuff, it has to be deflated and if the child has on his or her heat moisture exchange system, or "nosey," for humidification, it has to be taken off (Figure 7–6).

Depending on the age and overall ability of the child (including language and cognitive development), the clinician and eventually the parents or caregivers can briefly occlude the child's trach so he or she can vocalize. After the child is able to tolerate occlusion for voicing and other laryngeal functions (e.g., coughing), conferring with the medical team

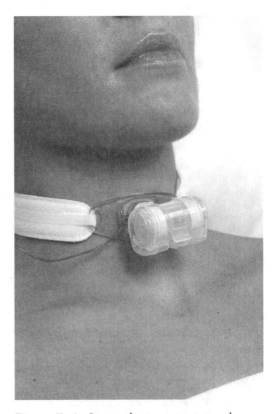

Figure 7–6. Bivona heat moisture exchange (HME) system. Image provided by Smiths-Medical. Used with permission.

to consider recommending the use of a speaking valve should be considered. Several criteria must be met in order for a child to use a speaking valve. Most importantly it requires that the child be able to fully and comfortably tolerate exhaling air through the larynx and upper airway for longer periods of time. When a speaking valve is in place, air is inhaled through the valve but exhaled through the upper airway. With the valve in place, transtracheal pressures must be maintained at less than 10 cm H_2O. Inability to maintain these lower pressures can result in elevated CO_2 levels, pulmonary injury, and discomfort (Brigger & Hartnick, 2009). Use of a speaking valve occurs only after a thorough team assessment that involves the physician, nurse, respiratory therapist and speech-language pathologist (SLP). The initial trials are always conducted with the child awake and under direct supervision. If the child is an inpatient, the respiratory therapist should be present during early trials to monitor the child's oxygen saturation (SaO_2), CO_2 levels, respiratory rate, heart rate, color, and overall respiratory comfort. If the patient is in an outpatient setting, the clinician should be sufficiently experienced with this population in order to make the required observations as well as seek any advice and assistance from the child's medical team.

Use of a speaking valve will afford the child the ability to develop voice and speech in a more natural fashion. A number of devices are commercially available. Some of the most widely used are the Passy-Muir® Tracheostomy and Ventilator Speaking Valves (Figure 7–7). These valves are patented, closed-position "no leak" valves designed to fit the 15-mm hub of most tracheostomy tubes. The valves open during inspiration, closing at the end of inspiration, redirecting all exhaled air through the oro- and nasopharynx, thereby permitting clear, uninterrupted speech production.

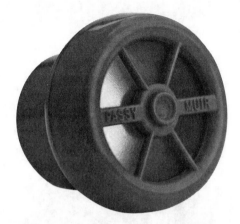

Figure 7–7. PMV® 2001 speaking valve used frequently by pediatric patients. Image courtesy of Passy-Muir, Inc., Irvine, CA. Used with permission.

When transitioning a child to a speaking valve such as the Passy-Muir Valve (PMV), often he or she will need retraining to overcome habitual chin dropping and to learn oral exhalation and nose blowing for the first time. Some children will develop behavioral tactics, such as breath holding, coughing off the valve, or taking it off, until they learn the benefits of communication. Depending on the child's individual diagnosis, medical status, and similar considerations, the PMV® can be worn virtually from infancy (Brigger & Hartnick, 2009) through the various communication stages permitting the baby the ability to babble, coo, laugh, and cry, all of which bring great satisfaction to their families (Figure 7–8).

According to the PMV literature and research done with adults, a speaking valve can also improve swallowing functions in children by returning oropharyngeal-laryngeal pressures to a non-trach condition and by permitting improved airway clearance through a stronger cough. The PMV creates a closed respiratory system that improves swallowing, reduces aspiration, facilitates secretion management, and reduces time for weaning and

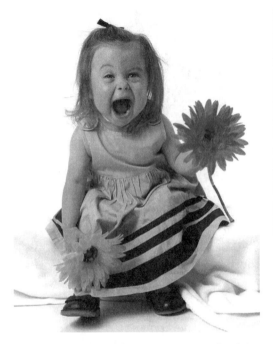

Clinical Note: Trachesotomy tube "plugging" or "capping" is often the last step before attempting removal of the tracheostomy tube (decannulation). All of the previously mentioned criteria for upper airway clearance must be met and the child must be able to tolerate adequate inhalation and exhalation to support ventilation and respiration through the upper airway for extended periods of time. A systematic approach to building tolerance (e.g., increases in time) for tracheostomy tube plugging is often implemented by the medical team. The plug is a cap that fits over the hub of the tracheostomy tube and prevents the inflow and outflow of air.

Figure 7–8. A pediatric patient with diagnosis of VATER, tracheomalacia, vocal fold paralysis, and chronic aspiration using the PMV® 2001 for speech, swallowing, and secretion management. Photo courtesy of Passy-Muir, Inc., Irvine, CA. Used with permission.

decannulation. The reduction of secretions occurs because the airflow facilitates their natural evaporation in the oral and nasal chambers. A closed respiratory system can improve the child's ability to cough and blow his nose and thus lower his susceptibility to bacterial infections (Passy-Muir, 2013).

Indications for use of a speaking valve like the PMV can include diagnoses of neuromuscular disease, quadriplegia, brain injury, tracheomalacia, mild tracheal and/or laryngeal stenosis, and bilateral vocal fold paralysis *without* significant airway obstruction, and conditions where patients are ventilator dependent or are emotionally or physically unable to tolerate tracheostomy tube plugging. Contraindications are for children who have

severe tracheal and/or laryngeal obstruction, gross aspiration, a laryngectomy, must maintain an inflated cuff, or are in an unconscious state (Woodnorth, 2004).

Decannulation

The ultimate goal of the medical team and the family is for the child to have the tracheostomy tube removed or to be decannulated. According to the most recent Clinical Consensus Statement, the stated criteria for decannulation include the child having been off the ventilator for at least 3 months, during which time he or she should demonstrate tolerance of respiratory infections without the ventilator and have no recurring aspiration events resulting in aspiration pneumonias. Visual inspection of the larynx should reveal at least one mobile true vocal fold (TVF) and no suprastomal granulation or severe subglottic stenosis. The child must be able to tolerate smaller tracheostomy tubes, capping, or complete occlusion of the trach through the day and eventually through the night, without any respiratory or related health consequence. Successful decannulation can take weeks, months, or longer. Factors that drive success include the sustained patency of the natural airway, airway protection, secretion management, pulmonary toileting needs, history of failed attempts, respiratory stability, and overall well-being of the child (Mitchell et al., 2012).

The long-term goal is to remove the tracheotomy tube; thus, when the child is stable, a permanent surgical solution such as airway reconstruction is needed to restore a viable upper airway (Cotton & McMurray, 1999; Hartley, Rutter, & Cotton, 2000; Lesperance & Zalzal, 1998). The success rates of decannulation following reconstruction procedures are reportedly high (Cotton & McMurray, 1999; Hartley et al., 1998). Unfortunately, long-term tracheostomy tube placement and the subsequent reconstruction procedures can result in voicing disturbances that disrupt the children's overall communication and potentially their quality of life (deAlarcon et al., 2009; Sell & MacCurtain, 1988).

Airway Reconstruction

The goal of pediatric airway reconstruction (AR) is to establish a patent laryngeal airway able to support ventilation/respiration, airway protection, and voicing and ultimately eliminate the need for a tracheostomy tube. Surgical AR procedures are performed to expand the laryngeal-tracheal airway and, in some cases, remove damaged areas (subglottic narrowing or stenosis). The most common AR procedure is a laryngotracheoplasty (LTP) with anterior and/or posterior costal cartilage graft (LTPACCG; LTPPCCG; LTPAPCCG). In these procedures a rib graft (taken from the same patient) is shaped to securely fit in the space between the cut surfaces of the anterior

or posterior (or both) cricoid lamina, expanding its circumference and thus the dimension of the subglottic airway. Damaged and thus narrow airway segments can extend up to the inferior aspect of the vocal folds. In such cases the area needing a graft may extend up to and include the inferior anterior aspect of the thyroid laminae (Figure 7–9). The anterior commissure of the larynx may need to be split and then surgically reapproximated. This process can affect the level of the TVFs and lead to altered vocal fold function.

In cases of higher grades of SGS (grades 3 and 4), a slightly different reconstruction procedure called cricotracheal resection (CTR) may be used (Myer, Cotton, & Schott, 1995; Monnier, Lang & Samvary, 2003). This procedure entails removing the anterior half of the cricoid lamina, as well as the mucosal covering of the posterior cricoid lamina. In addition, a number of the upper tracheal rings are completely removed. The upper and lower margins of the remaining airway are then surgically reconnected. The goal of this procedure is to completely remove the stenosed or narrow segment of the airway (Cotton, 2000; Hartley et al., 2000) (Figures 7–10 and 7–11).

Laryngotracheal and cricotracheal reconstruction procedures can be performed as a single or a double staged procedure (Gustafson et al., 2000). In a single staged procedure, the airway is reconstructed and the patient is intubated anywhere from 3 to 10 days. Double staged procedures are used in cases where prolonged stenting is required and/or there are multiple levels of airway obstruction. In children where a double staged procedure is required, a tracheostomy tube is placed below the level of reconstruction and a stent is placed traversing the reconstructed segment. The stents are removed after varying periods of time. The airway is then examined and, if deemed adequate, the tracheostomy tube is removed.

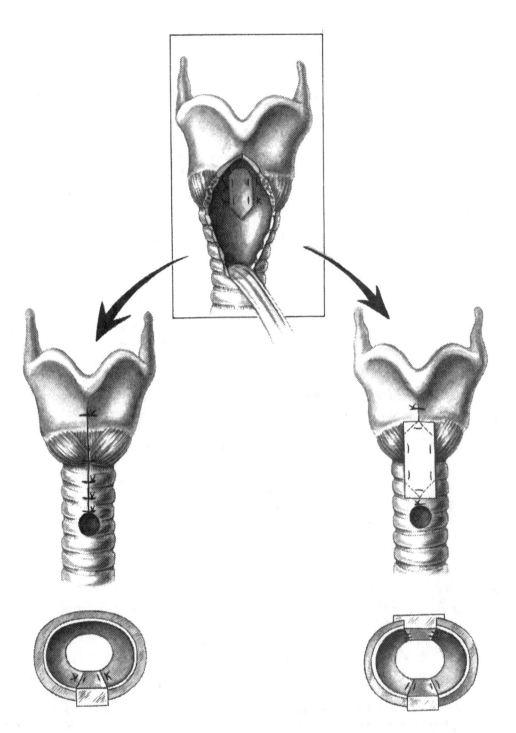

Figure 7–9. Combinations of augmentation sites are possible. The anterior and posterior costal cartilage grafts can be used alone or in combination. The augmentation technique is dependent on the stenois. From *The Pediatric Airway* by C. M. Myer III, R. T. Cotton, and S. R. Schott, 1995. Reprinted with permission from Lippincott, Williams & Wilkins.

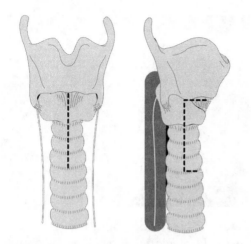

Figure 7–10. Cricotracheal resection. Image used with permission from the Department of Pediatric Otolaryngology, Head and Neck Surgery, Cincinnati Children's Hospital, Cincinnati, Ohio.

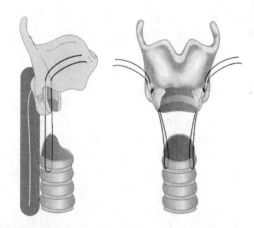

Figure 7–11. Cricotracheal reapproximation. Image used with permission from the Department of Pediatric Otolaryngology, Head and Neck Surgery, Cincinnati Children's Hospital, Cincinnati, Ohio.

Physical Findings and Voice Outcomes Post-Airway Reconstruction

The priority goal of AR is to restore a patent airway, but these necessary airway expansion procedures can have consequences for airway protection and voicing. Nearly 50% of children who undergo airway reconstruction are dysphonic (Baker et al., 2006; Kelchner et al., 2009). When the children are young, voice quality is typically a secondary concern for parents. It is more typical for parents to be relieved that their child no longer requires a tracheostomy. Concern over voice quality tends to emerge later, when the children become teenagers. That is when the children and their parents express new concerns about voice quality, specifically loudness (de Alarcón, 2012). These concerns stem from the child's social interactions with peers who may now call attention to the dysphonia and the difficulty the child has being heard and understood in noisy environments.

Voice outcomes postairway reconstruction include dysphonia marked by harshness, whisper, ventricular phonation, or inappropriate pitch. These qualities are due to postsurgical changes, including abnormal vocal fold mobility, a continued degree of SGS, anterior commissure blunting, and supraglottic compression (Figures 7–12 and 7–13; Baker et al., 2006; MacArthur, Kearns, & Healy, 1994). Etiology, preoperative grade of SGS, and surgery type also influence voice outcomes. Risk factors for poor voice outcomes include complete laryngofissure, posterior grafting, cricotracheal resection, and multiple airway reconstruction (Bailey, Clary, Penguilly, & Albert, 1995; Zalzal, Loomis, & Fisher, 1993). Patients with supraglottic and mixed glottic phonation will often have perceptually worse voice outcomes. Many of these patients have problems with glottic incompetence or glottic diastasis (always open glottis); thus, closure of the posterior glottis during phonation is often problematic (Zeitels, de Alarcon, Burns, Lopez-Guerra, & Hillman, 2011). There is a general consensus across investigations that children with lower grades of SGS (grades 1, 2), less complex medical histories, and single

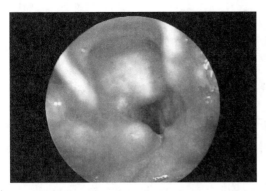

Figure 7–12. Possible physical findings post airway reconstruction. Image used with permission from the Center for Pediatric Voice Disorders, Cincinnati Children's Hospital, Cincinnati, Ohio.

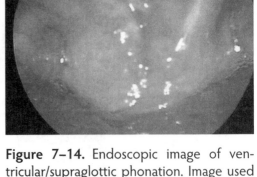

Figure 7–14. Endoscopic image of ventricular/supraglottic phonation. Image used with permission from the Center for Pediatric Voice Disorders, Cincinnati Children's Hospital, Cincinnati, Ohio.

stage surgical procedures demonstrate better voice quality (Smith, Marsh, Cotton & Myer, 1993; Zalzal, Loomis, Derkay, Murray & Thomsen, 1991).

If one or both of the TVFs and arytenoids are immobile, the child may compensate by compressing supraglottic structures. In the clinic setting, it is not uncommon to

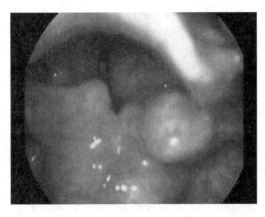

Figure 7–13. Possible physical findings post airway reconstruction. Image used with permission from the Center for Pediatric Voice Disorders, Cincinnati Children's Hospital, Cincinnati, Ohio.

observe the child use her ventricular folds for voicing as either an *obligatory* or *learned motor* compensation for poor glottic closure following surgery (Figure 7–14; Kelchner, Weinrich, Brehm, Tabangin, & de Alarcon, 2010). In some situations, it may be a prolapsed arytenoid that vibrates against the petiole of the epiglottis in order to generate sound. Eventually *habituated*, these variations of laryngeal function or alternate sources of vibration become chronic. See DVD: strobe sample 7 and 10.

Perceptually, these patients typically exhibit a range of dysphonia, but most are severe. Yet, voice quality and vibration patterns generated with supraglottic structures can be highly variable. Some children even achieve periodic vibration with their ventricular folds, suggesting an inherent flexibility and adaptability in the tissues used to make sound (Krival et al., 2007). This has important implications for treatment.

Following airway reconstruction, the required effort used to produce voice is also a common clinical complaint from parents and children alike. The children report symptoms of breathlessness, fatigue, and strain. These factors are observed by the parents as well. To examine the relationship between strain and site of vibration, Weinrich and colleagues (2007) examined the numeric values for airflow, estimated subglottal pressure, and perceptual rating of strain. This was a non-randomized prospective study that included children with glottic or supraglottic vibratory sources post AR. Of note, the participants were grouped according to site of vibration (50% were glottic; 50% were supraglottic) and the two groups were paired and matched by age and gender. Results revealed that expert perceptual ratings of strain, achieved by consensus, were significantly higher (meaning more severe) for participants with supraglottic versus glottic voicing. Although the mean airflow measures were higher for participants with glottic phonation and mean pressure measure was higher for those with supraglottic voicing, statistical significance was not found. Clinically, the increased values of airflow and pressure may reflect the physical complaints reported in patients with altered laryngeal mechanisms.

Voice Evaluation for the Child Pre- or Post-Airway Reconstruction

The child who is pre and/or post AR should participate in a comprehensive voice evaluation, similar to that described in Chapter 5. Importantly, the initial intake will pay special attention to the child's early history, including any and all airway management (including number and type of surgeries or other airway procedures), recent changes in medications, pulmonary status, swallowing and airway protection issues, nutritional status, developmental concerns, handicapping indices, and quality of life responses. Length and course of any intubation period and complications should be described in detail. Particular attention should be given to the child's communication development during intubation or with the tracheostomy in place. Capturing sufficient voiced segments for purposes of acoustic analysis can be challenging, and modifications to the full protocol may be required.

Many of these children are accustomed to being medically tested, therefore the process is not difficult or unfamiliar to them. As with any children, however, the ability to participate is dependent on factors related to their age, developmental level, behavior, and prior experiences. Care should always be taken to prepare the child and his or her parent for the entire process and provide warm-ups and opportunities to practice, so a best sample can be captured. The children often enjoy the time in the sound-treated booth (or "club house") using the microphone and watching the voice signal displays on the computer screen. Reassuring the child who has undergone numerous surgical procedures that the mask used to capture airflow is more like a "pilot's mask" rather than an anesthesia mask is a necessary step. Of note, some children who are post AR have "two voices" due to anatomic changes. That is, they may use supraglottic phonation for most conversation, but when prompted discover they can also generate some tones with their TVFs. When this is the case, attempts should be made to analyze both sources of voice.

The ability to accurately measure many of the acoustic and aerodynamic parameters in children post AR is important for evaluation protocol and treatment planning. Brehm and colleagues (2009) completed a retrospective examination of 100 children ages 3 to 17 years in regard to their ability to follow instructions and provide a sufficient speech sample for acoustic and aerodynamic analysis. In this study they examined the relationship of behavior (ability to cooperate with the task), age, and etiology to successfully conduct a full evaluation. Fifty-three of the 100 children met all of the inclusion criteria. Of those, 53% were able to complete the entire protocol without any modifications. Seventy-five percent of children were able to complete the vocal task for acoustic analysis, although a full analysis could not always be completed. Thirty-two percent of the children post AR produced a type I signal, which was appropriate for the measurement of average fundamental frequency (F_0). Sixty-four percent of the children were able to complete the entire aerodynamic portion of the evaluation protocol. There was a statistically significant correlation between age and the ability to complete the entire protocol. Not surprisingly, the younger, more developmentally delayed children had greater difficulty with the full protocol.

During the imaging portion of the voice evaluation, both the flexible and rigid endoscopes are used, as possible. In some instances an exam using high speed is conducted, especially if there are concerns about identifying the exact source(s) of vibration or tracking the voice signal source during stroboscopy. Once the images are captured, categorization of gross laryngeal function and the source of sound for voicing (indicating whether it is glottic, mixed glottic, and/or isolated supraglottic phonation) can be rated. Discrete parameters of vibratory behavior should also be rated as possible (via stroboscopic or high-speed examination) and will guide interventions.

Treatment of Dysphonia Following Airway Reconstruction

Treatment of dysphonia following AR is highly individualized. Decisions regarding treatment are usually based on observation of laryngeal function as seen on endoscopy, and the perceived severity of the voice disorder by the experts, parents, and child. There needs to be a thoughtful discussion as to what is achievable regarding voice improvement via surgical, medical, and behavioral therapies. Voice therapy can play a crucial role in both initial and postoperative management.

Medical and Surgical Treatment

Any surgical procedures performed with the goal of improving voice production will be tailored to the children's needs based on their specific post AR anatomy. Many children with postoperative AR dysphonia have a persistent glottic gap, typically in the posterior glottis. This gap is caused either by prior surgical intervention to improve the airway or by injury from intubation earlier in childhood. Initial surgical management may involve reversible procedures or procedures that have a minimal impact on respiration. One such procedure is temporary medialization laryngoplasty. This is similar to the procedure described earlier in Chapter 3 for the management of unilateral vocal fold paralysis; however, in children with postoperative AR dysphonia, both vocal folds (and sometimes one of the ventricular folds) may require medialization or augmentation. Following this surgery, there is typically more improvement in supraglottic versus glottic phonation. Improved approximation of the ventricular folds can result in improvements in loudness, clarity, and intelligibility. If the initial temporary procedure is successful, a more permanent procedure involving injection with autologous fat is often performed.

For children whose vocal folds are either misaligned or have a large anterior gap, the best correction is provided by an open surgical procedure to divide the anterior commissure to realign the vocal folds or close the anterior gap. For children with persistent posterior glottic opening, there are two surgical options, and both are generally reserved for children who have gone through puberty and have a fully grown airway. One option is to perform an endoscopic arytenoid flap. During this procedure, a portion of the aryepiglottic fold and the supraarytenoid tissue are rotated as a pediculed flap into the posterior glottis. This helps close off some of the posterior gap, leading to improved supraglottic phonation. A conceptually better option is the removal of a portion of the posterior cricoid plate, narrowing the posterior glottis. This can be performed through either an open or an endoscopic approach. The main risk of this procedure is the potential for postoperative airway obstruction. In view of this risk, families seldom choose this option.

Behavioral Therapy

To date, much of the evidence regarding voice therapy following pediatric AR is a combination of case-based reports and clinical anecdotes. The reason there are no group treatment studies is that children who are post AR present with a variety of airway injuries and surgical histories. Controlling all the possible variables in order to test a controlled intervention is a challenge, as is access to these children after they leave the hospital. Management and follow-up care of these children often take place at multiple institutions. The child may start with local care, then be referred to regional or national centers for more complex care, and then return back to local care, which includes the public schools.

As described in Chapter 6, early goals of therapy are focused on educating the child and his or her parent about how to best care for the voice. Gathering as much data as possible from the initial assessment team is essential for the treating clinician. Assessing the child's (and parent/caregiver's) motivation to enroll in voice therapy must also be determined, as sometimes these children and their families are not up to the task of more intervention. The treating clinician can share insights regarding the social, educational, and occupational challenges of having a lifelong severe dysphonia as they determine that the family and patient are prepared to receive that information.

If the treating clinician knows that a child is using supraglottic phonation, he may conclude that the child will have a very limited ability to change his or her voice quality. However, with direction and guidance, many of these children are able to manipulate their supraglottic voice quality. The treating clinician should probe for the best sound and one that uses the least amount of effort. Interestingly many children actually lead the way with this task through vocal play. With guidance they can discover their own ability to control the dynamics of their sound source and ultimately their intelligibility, which is often aided by improvements in loudness and inflection. Using "priming gestures," as described in Chapter 6, is an excellent tool to help the children make discoveries about how they can control their voices.

Children post AR commonly require high subglottic pressures to initiate and sustain voicing, resulting in increased effort and strain. By using a semioccluded or modified resonant voice type exercises, the work of voicing can be reduced and the use of modified vocal function exercises can help the children explore their vocal agility. As with all therapy, successful carryover of techniques into connected speech can be a challenge. Even with successful voice quality improvement, it is not uncommon for children to be reticent about using a "new" or different-sounding voice in public. See DVD: Challenging Case.

A highly structured, dose-driven therapy that includes a family-centered home program is needed for success. Treatments started at specialized centers should transition smoothly to local care. It is important for the specialized voice teams to seek and develop relationships with local private and or school-based SLPs and to offer their support throughout therapy. In the near future, this type of therapy and support should be available through a telehealth model of care.

Pediatric Laryngectomy

Symptoms and Causes

Up to 5% of all childhood malignancies originate in the head and neck; however, as a procedure, the need for pediatric laryngectomy is rare. Soft tissue sarcomas and benign but locally aggressive (peripheral) neural tumors that grow and obstruct the laryngeal airway are examples of disease processes that may necessitate a full or partial laryngectomy (Garabédian, Ducroz, Ayache, & Triglia 1999; McDermott, Raj, Glaholm, Pearman, & Macnamara, 2000). In children, detection of a malignant disease in the hypopharynx or larynx may be delayed due to delay of significant onset of symptoms (dysphagia and dysphonia) and the child's inability to clearly report them. In a child, as in adults, the presence of any new or progressive dysphonia without other respiratory symptoms dictates the urgent need for an otolaryngologic examination. Advanced symptoms might include stridor, change in feeding or swallowing abilities, report of pain, nutritional compromise, and palpable masses and lymph nodes.

Treatment

Nowhere is the collaborative approach to treatment more essential than it is with the child who requires a total laryngectomy. A total laryngectomy involves removal of the entire larynx (and possibly adjacent tissue and lymph nodes), resulting in a complete separation of the aerodigestive tract, permanently moving the airway to the neck, and a loss of the laryngeal source of voicing. The surgeon and his or her team's decision to perform a laryngectomy will come at the end of a long medical evaluation and after all other treatment options have been exhausted.

Postoperative communication management and support for the child will require the coordinated efforts of hospital-based, outpatient, and school SLPs. When caring for adults, the standard course of care is to provide preoperative counseling, which usually reviews the surgery, its subsequent anatomic changes, and the impact on communication. However, this option may not be possible for the family of a child, either for timing or for emotional reasons. At minimum, the anticipated course of postoperative care, including communication options, should be discussed with the family (and the child if age appropriate) prior to surgery. The child will likely already have a tracheostomy tube and be accustomed to communicating by either finger occluding it or using a speaking valve, so the concept of an alternate airway will be familiar. Importantly, the inpatient SLP needs to have a familiar and uncomplicated means by which the child can communicate with the nursing staff and family postoperatively, as soon as the child is medically able.

Planning for the child's near- and long-term communication needs will depend on what other medical-surgical treatments may be necessary. Once additional treatment options are known, the SLP can confer with the medical team and family to discuss whether esophageal speech, use of an artificial larynx, or use of a voice prosthesis should be the long-term communication mode of choice. Esophageal speech is the most independent means by which to communicate postlaryngectomy, but it is a technique that can be difficult both to teach and to learn. Practicing air injection techniques after swallowing a carbonated beverage is a technique used by adults. For the child, friendly competitions with siblings and

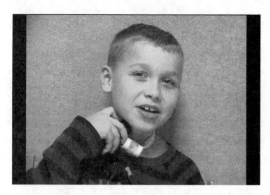

Figure 7–15. Child post laryngectomy using electrolarynx.

friends to "burp talk" can be helpful. An artificial larynx may be the most immediate usable option. The known drawbacks include the nonnatural mechanical sound and the need to hold it in place (Figure 7–15). For multiple reasons in the younger child, use of a voice prosthesis is not likely to be the first option. Placement of a voice prosthesis requires an additional tracheoesophageal puncture surgery and the custom manufacture of a pediatric voice prosthesis.

To fully support the child and his or her family, extra care should be taken for the seamless transfer of care from the hospital-based clinicians to the school or community SLPs. Consulting local adult voice care SLPs who have extensive experience in laryngectomy care should enhance available intervention approaches.

Paradoxical Vocal Fold Dysfunction

Paradoxical vocal fold dysfunction (PVFD) is an involuntary adduction of the vocal folds during the inspiratory phase of breathing that results in an obstruction of the airway. This paradoxical movement of the vocal folds can be precipitated by factors related to physical exercise, laryngeal hyperreactivity, or emotions. In more severe episodes, the supraglottic structures may also adduct during inspiration, leading to a greater degree of obstruction. Many names have been given to this disorder, including but not limited to vocal fold dysfunction (VCD), paradoxical vocal cord movement (PVCM), and episodic paroxysmal laryngospasm (EPL). This disorder is most commonly seen in patients between the ages of 10 and 40 years (Kuppersmith, Rosen, & Wiatrak, 1993).

Symptoms and Causes

The symptoms associated with PVFD are generally episodic and intermittent, being triggered by a variety of stimulants. PVFD is often misdiagnosed as asthma or chronic cough due to the similarity of symptoms. Creating even greater difficulty in diagnosis, PVFD often co-occurs in patients who have diagnosed asthma. Common characteristics observed during an episode of PVFD are neck or upper chest tightness and inspiratory stridor. Patients also report dyspnea (or breathlessness) or air hunger, coughing, and voice change. Wheezing is also reported in some patients, as frequently the obstruction of the airway carries over to the expiratory phase of breathing.

The most commonly cited cause of PVFD throughout the literature discussing this disorder is an underlying psychological disturbance. In fact this disorder was first described in the literature as Munchausen stridor (Patterson, Schatz, & Houton, 1974). However, more recent literature suggests that in some cases there are underlying medical conditions as the cause, such as LPR. In fact, 36% to 95% of children with PVFD have laryngeal tissue changes consistent with LPR (Powell et al., 2000). Although rare, neurologic disorders such as a brainstem tumor may cause paradoxing of the vocal folds (Mashcka et al., 1997).

Diagnosis

As stated above, the diagnosis of PVFD is challenging because the symptoms mimic other respiratory disorders, and asthma actually has been reported to co-occur with PVFD 50% of the time (Newman, Mason, & Schmaling, 1995). Diagnosis of this disorder is often completed by a team of professionals, including a pediatric otolarynogologist, pediatric pulmonologist, and SLP. Attempts are made by the evaluation team to view evidence of paradoxical activity during a laryngeal examination (using a flexible endoscope). Some patients with this disorder have a consistent slight adduction of the vocal folds even when asymptomatic that can be viewed during a laryngeal examination (Treole, Trudeau, & Forrest, 1999). Often, in order to observe any paradoxical movement, the evaluation team must attempt to elicit a stimulating event such as having the child walk up and down stairs or other strenuous physical activity. In some centers, a flexible examination might be performed while the child is walking/running on a treadmill to elicit a high level of exercise in a controlled environment. There are many cases in which the paradoxical movement is never observed during the clinical evaluation. In these cases, the diagnosis of PVFD may be made as a "diagnosis of exclusion." When evaluating a child who appears to have symptoms of PVFD, it is important to consider all other causes of airway obstruction, including vocal fold paralysis, recurrent respiratory papilloma, asthma, etc.

Treatment

Differential diagnosis of PVFD often extends into the treatment phase, as investigation of the triggers and stimulants for episodes may take longer with some children. Children are often encouraged to keep a journal of events involving stress, food, and environment that trigger episodes. Education of parents and children regarding the normal and abnormal function of the larynx during episodes is a good first step in treatment. When possible, allowing the parent and child to view the laryngeal exam and to see paradoxical vocal fold movement may be helpful. The course of therapy for a patient with PVFD should generally be short. Often patients are seen for as few as one or two sessions.

Several published articles provide an overview of the disorders as well as very concrete treatment plans for patients. One such article, by Adrianopoulos, Gallivan, and Gallivan (2000), outlines a three-phase therapy program that could easily be adapted for children. The three phases include: (1) a differential diagnosis and obtaining of baseline data, (2) multidisciplinary management, and (3) carryover. The *multidisciplinary management* phase involves behavior management using motor learning theories and neurolinguistic reprogramming. The process involves identifying behaviors and developing strategies to improve function. Respiratory training techniques such as focus on abdominal breathing, panting, and pursed lip inhalation are taught in this phase as well. The *carryover* phase promotes independence and self-awareness to use the strategies learned in the presence of a stimulus.

Sandage and Zelazny (2004) also provide a multistep behavioral and exercise program that can be used with children that focuses on progressive relaxation techniques, abdominal breathing, and recovery exercises to be used when an episode of paradoxing occurs. Their published article provides an extensive description of these exercises in the appendices.

There are currently two published case studies examining the use of an inspiratory muscle strength training program in adolescent athletes with PVFD (Mathers-Schmidt & Brilla, 2005; Ruddy et al., 2004). Both of these reports found decreased perceptions of dyspnea during exercise and an eventual complete elimination of paradoxical episodes during sports activities. This is a promising area of treatment; however, much more supporting evidence is needed. Research in patients with PVFD is very challenging, as there are many presentations of the disorder as well as causes/triggers.

Puberphonia

Puberphonia is a disorder characterized by maintenance of a high-pitched voice by a male who is progressing through puberty. In addition to a high-pitched quality, the voice is often breathy with low volume. Other terms for this disorder include mutational falsetto and pubescent falsetto.

Symptoms and Causes

Commonly, this disorder is thought to be caused by an underlying psychological disorder related to problems accepting a new, lower male voice, emotional/social immaturity, and gender identification concerns. An adolescent male who is exhibiting symptoms of puberphonia should undergo a medical evaluation, as other causes have been identified such as hearing loss, delayed maturation of laryngeal structures due to an endocrine disorder, and neuromuscular control issues.

Diagnosis

Common findings on laryngeal examination of an adolescent with puberphonia generally "fit" with the voice quality. Often laryngeal structures appear normal and appropriately sized for the patient; however, glottal closure may be incomplete, with accompanying hyperfunction of laryngeal structures. Hyperfunction may be evidenced by a higher laryngeal position and tension/compression of supraglottic structures. In addition to the high-pitched, breathy quality described above, the lack of glottic closure can cause difficulty with speaking loudly or over background noise and may lead to vocal fatigue.

Treatment

Management techniques for puberphonia include the use of laryngeal massage therapy and reduction of tension during speech (see Chapter 6 for a special note about the use of laryngeal massage in children). Visual biofeedback techniques with specialized speech software such as Real-Time Pitch from KayPENTAX using a Visi-Pitch allows the clinician to mark acceptable frequency ranges for speech productions. Electroglottography was also used as a biofeedback tool in one study with adolescents with puberphonia with significant hearing loss (Chernobelsky, 2002). Often in therapy, the appropriate voice may be "found" with the patient and it can be used quite easily in unstructured conversation; however, the use of this "new" voice amongst certain family members or peers may require great support and advice from the treating clinician.

Muscle Tension Dysphonia: An Overview

MTD is a disorder of the larynx characterized by general excessive muscular activity in the head and neck. Descriptions of this disorder and reports of cases in the literature relate primarily to adults. The underlying cause of the disorder is typically related to stress, high workloads, and high vocal demands.

Although there are no current reports in the literature of large numbers of children having MTD or even in clinical sites that see many children, features of this disorder can occur in children who are exposed to high levels of stress for a variety of reasons.

Laryngeal examination in patients with this disorder typically reveals normally appearing laryngeal structures; however, during phonation, there can be hyperfunction of the entire larynx (vocal folds and supraglottic structures). On stroboscopy, a decrease in the amplitude of vocal fold vibration can be observed. Large glottal gaps to incomplete closure of the vocal folds during phonation may also be seen. Common voice quality characteristics include strain and an abnormally high pitch. In cases in which there is incomplete vocal fold closure, extreme breathiness or aphonia may be the primary vocal parameter.

Treatment of this disorder focuses on general head and neck relaxation techniques as well as the potential for laryngeal massage therapy (again, see the section of Chapter 6 regarding laryngeal massage in children). There is one documented study of effective therapy in children with MTD in the literature ($n = 8$) in which biofeedback and self-awareness task regarding tension were employed as well as easy onsets for initiating speech (Lee & Son, 2005). According to the authors, using these techniques improved voice quality in these children.

Putting It All Together: Case Summaries

Case Summary 1. Patient: Sam (Pediatric Laryngectomy)

History

Sam was a 7-year-old male with a diagnosis of inflammatory myofibroblastic tumor of the larynx and hypopharynx/upper esophagus. After repeated attempts to manage the disease in his neck (during which time Sam was trached), it became necessary for Sam to undergo a total laryngo (upper) esophagectomy. Prior to the surgical procedure, Sam's family met with the SLP to discuss implications for long-term communication and swallowing issues. Several key points were stressed, including the fact that the vibrating mechanism of the voice would be permanently removed. The family needed to hear these explanations multiple times before they realized the long-term implications for voice. Understanding and grasping the permanence of losing natural voice is not easily appreciated in one conversation.

Alternative communication for the immediate postoperative period, as well as long-term options, were also discussed with Sam and his family. As Sam was only just beginning to read, we introduced a simple communication board (with pictures denoting common needs), a yes/no response system, and a clicker, so he could signal a need to communicate. Sam also practiced with simple devices (e.g., magic slate) and an iPad. Knowing that the details of our preop conversations might be lost given the overwhelming health care decisions and issues at hand, the voice specialist and inpatient SLPs conferred on strategies to reinforce all information during the immediate postoperative period.

Summary of Treatment

The size and extent of the tumor required Sam to undergo a total laryngectomy, partial (hypo) pharyngectomy, and upper esophagectomy. A radial forearm free-flap was used to rebuild the upper esophagus. A gastric tube (G-tube) was placed for nutrition. While an inpatient, Sam's initial postoperative course was rocky, which resulted in a prolonged stay. Although his mood varied (depending on his overall comfort and stress levels), Sam used his communication options well. As soon as his neck was sufficiently healed and some of the swelling diminished, the electrolarynx was introduced. Initial placement of the electrolarynx included Sam's cheeks and directly under his chin. These early sessions focused on obtaining the best placement, articulation, and timing of short connected speech segments. Prior to discharge, the family received extensive education from nursing, respiratory therapy, nutrition, and the SLP regarding all elements of his care at home. Sam was discharged home with a TruTone electrolarynx as well as his other communication devices. By her own choice, Sam's public school SLP was extensively involved in his care throughout the course of his hospitalization. This significantly aided his long-term communication recovery.

Continuation of Care

Upon discharge, a TRACOE twist laryngeal tube was placed in the stoma, and a heat moisture exchange system (an artificial nose, or "nosey") for warming, humidification, and filtering purposes is always worn. Alternate laryngeal tubes are used and accommodations are made when he participates in sports. He returns to the medical center at regular intervals for a full evaluation of his swallowing, nutritional, communication, airway, and esophageal functions. He required a number of esophageal dilations to permit improved bolus flow of solid consistencies. After some initially slow progress, Sam is now able to maintain all of his nutritional needs via an unrestricted full oral diet. It is important to note that he receives excellent care at home.

Using a collaborative approach among his family, school, and hospital-based SLPs, Sam has learned to effectively communicate using his electrolarynx. Secure teleconferencing is used periodically to connect his home and hospital-based SLP team. Once best placement for the electrolarynx was determined, his intelligibility significantly improved. With direction from his school SLP and by his own talents, Sam quickly adapted the precision of his articulation and the timing of his phrasing, although having to hold the electrolarynx during any speech and physical activity remains a problem. Adaptation of an adult device to permit him to use the electrolarynx hands free is under way.

Sam is also learning esophageal speech under the close guidance of his school SLP, who also happens to be a clinician who can effectively instruct this communication method. Using carbonated drinks and with motivation from his siblings, he continues to make progress with injection techniques and is up to one or two word combinations. Currently any contemplation of an additional surgery for a tracheoesophageal puncture is postponed until he grows, matures, and remains disease free. Socially, Sam continues to make significant progress. The school personnel embrace his health issues and recovery by providing opportunities for him to build his social and communicative confidence. He fully participates in all types of school and community activities, including making announcements over the school PA system and participating in sports (see DVD: 2 videos for Sam).

Case Summary 2. Patient: Katie (Paradoxical Vocal Fold Dysfunction)

History

Katie was a 13-year-old female enrolled in the seventh grade. She was an outstanding student academically and participated in several school sports. During the middle of her soccer season, she had a fairly significant upper respiratory illness and her pediatrician recommended several medications, including a nasal spray. The nasal spray sparked a bad cough reaction and she experienced many coughing episodes long after she recovered from her illness. A few weeks later, she began feeling very short of breath during a soccer game and her teammates and coach could suddenly hear her breathing very "noisily." She was taken out of the game and sat on the sidelines for quite some time before she was breathing without stridor again. The shortness of breath began to occur at every soccer practice, and Katie reported to her parents that her neck felt very tight and she was very scared during the episodes.

Voice Evaluation

Katie was seen for a voice evaluation by an SLP and pediatric otolaryngologist at a children's hospital near her home. Flexible endoscopy revealed normal-appearing laryngeal structures during breathing at rest and during phonation; however, no paradoxical episodes were observed. The SLP took Katie to a nearby hallway and set of stairs and had her complete a moderate level of walking and climbing. Despite this attempt at eliciting an episode, one could never be produced during the examination time. The only abnormal finding on the examination was some red, inflamed tissue in the interarytenoid space. The otolaryngologist prescribed a proton pump inhibitor to address the possible effects of acid reflux disease on the paradoxical episodes. Despite the fact that no evidence of laryngeal paradoxing was observed during the examination, a diagnosis of PVFD was made (as a diagnosis of exclusion) and Katie was referred for voice therapy.

Summary of the Treatment Procedures

During the first therapy session, the SLP reviewed a recording of the laryngeal examination with Katie and her parents to discuss the position of the glottis during breathing and speaking. The SLP described what likely was happening during paradoxical episodes. Katie was taught relaxation exercises and breathing exercises that focused on the reduction of muscle tension in the neck, throat, and upper chest area. She was also taught a recovery breathing exercise that consisted of three quick sniffs through the nose or inhaled through pursed lips with a long exhale. Additionally, due to symptoms and previous evidence of acid reflux, dietary precautions and discussion of how to take the prescribed medication were provided. The SLP asked Katie to keep a simple diary of symptoms, the effectiveness of the recovery technique, and her diet over the next week.

Treatment Outcomes

Katie returned one week later and was very excited to report the use and success of the recovery technique during soccer practice, when she had experienced several paradoxical episodes. Her diary indicated that she had not consistently taken her prescribed proton pump inhibitor, and the SLP provided additional education about reflux disease, emphasizing that patients often do not experience any noticeable symptoms. A third session was not scheduled, but rather the SLP told Katie that she would call her in a week to see if she was continuously able to use the recovery technique during soccer games and practice. During that follow-up phone call, Katie reported that she had had only one paradoxical episode in the previous week, which had occurred toward the end of a competitive game. She had been able to successfully use the recovery technique and the episode had quickly passed. The SLP made one more follow-up call 2 weeks later and Katie and her parents reported a complete cessation of symptoms. Katie was discharged from therapy at that time with the assurance that she could call the treating SLP in the future if she had further difficulty.

Conclusion

This final chapter reviewed key management issues for children with complex airway and low incidence (but high importance) voice conditions. Caring for these children requires a focused understanding of anatomy and physiology of the laryngeal mechanism and how airway injuries and needed treatments can impact the child's voice for a lifetime. SLPs, whether in medical, private, or public school settings, have to work closely and collaboratively with their medical colleagues in order to best care for these children. Case and care examples for two such children were provided at the end of the chapter. Additional examples and demonstrations can be found on the accompanying DVD.

References

Adrianopoulos, M. V., Gallivan, G. J., & Gallivan, K. H. (2000). PVCM, PVCD, EPL, and irritable larynx syndrome: What are we talking about and how do we treat it? *Journal of Voice, 14,* 607–618.

American Lung Association. (2013). Respiratory distress syndrome and broncho pulmonary dysplasia. Retrieved from http://www.action.lung.org/site/

Bailey, C. M., Clary, R. A,, Penguilly, A., Albert, D. M. (1995). Voice quality following laryngotracheal construction. *International Journal of Pediatric Otorhinolaryngology 32*(Suppl.), S93–S95.

Baker, S., Kelchner, L., Weinrich, B., Lee, L., Willging, P., Cotton, R., & Zur, K. (2006). Voice assessment and treatment considerations in pediatric laryngotracheal stenosis. *Journal of Voice, 20*(4), 631–641.

Brehm, S. B., Weinrich, B., Zieser, M., Kelchner, L., Middendorf, J., Elluru, R., de Alarcon, A. (2009). Aerodynamic and acoustic assessment in children following airway reconstruction: An assessment of feasibility. *International Journal of Pediatric Otorhinolaryngology, 73,* 1019–23.

Brigger, M. T., & Hartnick, C. J. (2009). Drilling speaking valves: A modification to improve vocalization in tracheostomy dependent children. *Laryngoscope, 119*(1), 176–179.

Carron, J. D., Derkay, C. S., Strope, G. L., Nosonchuk, J. E., & Darrow, D. H. (2000). Pediatric tracheotomies: changing indications and outcomes. *Laryngoscope, 110*(7), 1099–1104.

Centers for Disease Control. (2013). Preterm birth. Retrieved September 27, 2013, from http://www.cdc.gov/reproductivehealth/Maternal InfantHealth/PretermBirth.htm.

Chernobelsky, S. (2002). The use of electroglottography in the treatment of deaf adolescents with puberphonia. *Logopedics, Phoniatrics, & Vocology, 27,* 63–65.

Cordeiro, A. M. G., Fernandes, J. C., & Troster, E. J. (2004). Possible risk factors associated with moderate or severe airway injuries in children who underwent endotracheal intubation. *Pediatric Critical Care Medicine, 5,* 364–368.

Cotton, R. T. (2000). Management of subglottic stenosis. *Otolaryngology Clinics of North America, 33,* 111–130.

Cotton, R. T., & McMurray, J. S. (1999). Laryngotracheal stenosis. New perspectives. *Pediatric Pulmonology. Suppl. 18,* 64–66.

da Silva, O., & Stevens, D. (1999). Complications of airway management in very-low-birth-weight infants. *Biology of the Neonate, 75,* 40–45.

de Alarcón, A. (2012).Voice outcomes after pediatric airway reconstruction. *Laryngoscope, 122*(Suppl. 4), S84–S86.

de Alarcón, A., Brehm, S. B., Kelchner, L. N., Meinzen-Derr, J., Middendorf, J., & Weinrich, B. (2009). Comparison of pediatric voice handicap index scores with perceptual voice analysis in patients following airway reconstruction. *Annals of Otology Rhinology and Laryngology, 118,* 581–586.

Dikeman, K. J., & Kazandjian, M. S. (2003). *Communication and swallowing management of tracheostomized and ventilator-dependent patients (2nd ed.).* New York, NY: Thomson-Delmar Learning

Downing, G. J., & Kilbride, H. W. (1995). Evaluation of airway complications in high-risk preterm infants: application of flexible fiberoptic airway endoscopy. *Pediatrics, 95,* 567–572.

Elpern, E. H., Borkgren Okonek, M., Bacon, M., Gerstrung, C., & Skrzynski, M. (2000). Effect of the Passy-Muir tracheostomy speaking valve on pulmonary aspiration in adults. *Heart and Lung, 29,* 287–293.

Garabédian, E. N., Ducroz, V., Ayache, D., & Triglia, J. M. (1999). Results of partial laryngectomy for benign neural tumors of the larynx in children. *Annals of Otology Rhinology and Laryngology, 108,* 666–671.

Gustafson, L. M., Hartley, B. E., Liu, J. H., Link, D. T., Chadwell, J., Koebbe, C., . . . Cotton, R. T. (2000). Single-stage laryngotracheal reconstruction in children: A review of 200 cases. *Otolaryngology-Head and Neck Surgery, 123,* 430–434.

Hartley, B. E., Rutter, M. J., Cotton, R. T. (2000). Crichotracheal resection as a primary procedure for laryngotracheal stenosis in children. *International Journal of Pediatric Otorhinolaryngology, 54,* 133–136.

Jiang, D., & Morrison, G. A. (2003). The influence of long-term tracheostomy on speech and language development in children. *International Journal of Pediatric Otorhinolaryngology, 67*(Suppl. 1), S217–S220.

Kelchner, L. N., Brehm, S. B., Weinrich, B., Middendorf, J., deAlarcon, A., Levin, L., & Elluru, R. (2009). Perceptual evaluation of severe pediatric voice disorders: Rater reliability using the Consensus Auditory Perceptual Evaluation of Voice. *Journal of Voice, 24*(4), 441–449

Kelchner, L. Weinrich, B., Brehm, S., Tabangin, M., de Alarcon, A. (2010). Characterization of supraglottic phonation in children post airway reconstruction. *Annals of Otology, Rhinology and Laryngology, 119,* 383–390.

Krival, K., Kelchner, L., Weinrich, B., Baker, S., Lee, L., Middendorf, J., & Zur, K. (2007). Vibratory source, vocal quality, and fundamental frequency following pediatric laryngotracheal reconstruction. *International Journal of Pediatric Otorhinolaryngology, 71,* 1261–1269.

Kuppersmith, R., Rosen, D. S., & Wiatrak, B. J. (1993). Functional stridor in adolescents. *Journal of Adolescent Health, 14,* 166–171.

Lee, W., Koltai, P., Harrison, M., Elumalai, A., Bourdakos, D., Davis, . . . Connor, J. (2002). Indications for tracheotomy in the pediatric intensive care unit population. *Archives of Otolaryngology-Head and Neck Surgery, 128,* 1249–1252.

Lee, E. K., & Son, Y. I. (2005). Muscle tension dysphonia in children: Voice characteristics and outcome of voice therapy. *International Journal of Pediatric Otorhinolaryngology, 69,* 911–917.

Lesperance, M. M., & Zalzal, G. H. (1998). Laryngotracheal stenosis in children. *European Archives of Otorhinolaryngology, 255,* 12–17.

MacArthur, C. J., Kearns, G. H., Healy, G. B. (1994). Voice quality after laryngotracheal reconstruction. *Archives of Otolaryngology-Head and Neck Surgery, 120,* 641–647.

March of Dimes. (2013). Prematurity research. Retrieved from http://www.marchofdimes.com/research/prematurityresearch.html.

Maschka, D. A., Bauman, N. M., McCray, P. B., Jr., Hoffman, H. T., Karnell, M. P., & Smith, R. J. H. (1997). A classification scheme for paradoxical vocal cord motion. *Laryngoscope, 107,* 1429–1435.

Mathers-Schmidt, B. A., & Brilla, L. R. (2005). Inspiratory muscle training in exercise-induced paradoxical vocal fold motion. *Journal of Voice, 19,* 635–644.

McDermott A., Raj, P., Glaholm, J., Pearman, K., & Macnamara, M. (2000). De novo laryngeal carcinoma in childhood. *Journal of Laryngology and Otology, 114,* 293–295.

Mitchell, R. B., Hussey, H. M., Setzen, G., Jacobs, I. N., Nussenbaum, B., Dawson, C., . . . Merati, A. (2012). Clinical consensus statement: Tracheostomy care. *Otolaryngology-Head and Neck Surgery, 148,* 6–20.

Monnier, P., Lang, F., & Samvary, M. (2003). Partial cricotracheal resection for pediatric subglottic stenosis: a single institution's experience in 60 cases. *European Archives of Oto-rhinolaryngology, 260,* 295–297.

Myer, C. M., Cotton, R. T., & Shott, S. R. (1995). *The pediatric airway: An interdisciplinary approach.* Philadelphia, PA: Lippincott.

Myer, C. M., O'Connor, D. M., Cotton, R. T. (1994). Proposed grading system for subglottic stenosis based on endotracheal tube sizes. *Annals of Otology, Rhinology and Laryngology. 103,* 319–323.

Newman, K. B., Mason, U. G., & Schmaling, K. B. (1995). Clinical features of vocal cord dysfunction. *American Jourtory Critical Care Medicine, 152,* 1382–1386.

Norman, V., Louw, B., & Kritzinger, A. (2007). Incidence and description of dysphagia in infants and toddlers with tracheostomies: A retrospective review. *International Journal of Pediatric Otorhinolaryngology, 71,* 1087–1092.

Passy-Muir (2013). Clinical and product information. Retrieved from http://passy-muir.com /education

Patterson, R., Schatz, M., & Horton, M. (1974). Munchausen's stridor: Non-organic laryngeal obstruction. *Clinical Allergy, 4,* 307–310.

Pereira, K. D., MacGregor, A. R., McDuffie, C. M., & Mitchell, R. B. (2003). Tracheostomy in preterm infants, current trends. *Archives Otolaryngology-Head and Neck Surgery, 129,* 1268–1271.

Powell, D. M., Karanfilov, B. I., Beechler, K. B., Treole, K., Trudeau, M. D., & Forrest, L. A. (2000). Paradoxical vocal fold dysfunction in juveniles. *Archives of Otolaryngology-Head and Neck Surgery, 126,* 29–34.

Ruddy, B. H., Davenport, P., Baylor, J., Lehman, J., Baker, S., & Sapienza, C. (2004). Inspiratory muscle strength training with behavioral therapy in a case of a rower with presumed exercise-induced paradoxical vocal-fold dysfunction. *International Journal of Pediatric Otorhinolaryngology, 68,* 1327–1332.

Sandage, M. J., & Zelazny, S. K. (2004). Paradoxical vocal fold motion in children and adolescents. *Language, Speech, and Hearing Services in Schools, 35,* 353–362.

Sell, D., & MacCurtain, F. (1988). Speech and language development in children with acquired subglottic stenosis. *Journal of Laryngology and Otology,* (Suppl. 17), 35–38.

Simon, B. M., Fowler, S. M., & Handler, S. D. (1983). Communication development in young children with long-term tracheostomies: preliminary report. *International Journal of Pediatric Otorhinolaryngology, 6,* 37–50.

Smith, M. E., Marsh, J. H., Cotton, R. T., & Myer, C. M. (1993). Voice problems after pediatric laryngotracheal reconstruction: Videolaryngostroboscopic, acoustic, and perceptual assessment. *International Journal of Pediatric Otorhinolaryngology, 25,* 173–181.

Treole, K., Trudeau, M. D., & Forrest, L. A. (1999). Endoscopic and stroboscopic description of adults with paradoxical vocal fold dysfunction. *Journal of Voice, 13,* 143–152.

Walner, D. L., Loewen, M. S., & Kimura, R. E. (2001). Neonatal subglottic stenosis—incidence and trends. *Laryngoscope, 111,* 48–51.

Weinrich, B., Baker, S. Kelchner, L., Middendorf, J., Elluru, R., & Zur, K. (2007). Examination of aerodynamic measures and strain by vibratory source. *Archives of Otolaryngology-Head and Neck Surgery, 136,* 455–458.

Woodnorth, G. (2004). Assessing and managing medically fragile children: Tracheostomy and ventilatory support. *Language, Speech, and Hearing Services in the Schools, 35,* 363–372.

Zalzal, G. H., Loomis, S. R., Derkay, C. S., Murray, S. L., & Thomsen, J. (1991). Vocal quality of decannulated children following laryngeal reconstruction. *Laryngoscope, 101,* 425–429.

Zalzal, G. H., Loomis, S. R., & Fisher, M. (1993). Laryngeal reconstruction in children: assessment of vocal quality. *Archives of Otolaryngology-Head and Neck Surgery, 119,* 504–507.

Zeitels, S. M., de Alarcon, A., Burns, J. A., Lopez-Guerra, G., & Hillman, R. E. (2011). Posterior glottic diastasis: Mechanically deceptive and often overlooked. *Annals of Otology, Rhinology and Laryngology, 120,* 71–80.

Appendix A. Supplement on Wound Healing and the Vocal Folds

Keiko Ishikawa

Wound Healing and the Vocal Folds

As reviewed in Chapter 4, a variety of vocal fold pathologies can result in dysphonia. Some types of pathology such as vocal fold nodules, polyps, vocal process granuloma, and vocal fold scar are secondary to injury of the mucosa. Patients may receive voice therapy alone as treatment, whereas others undergo phonosurgery to resect pathologic tissue. The patient often receives voice therapy after the surgery, and in some cases therapy both precedes and follows surgery. In any of the situations, the clinicians' task is to restore optimal vocal function while promoting healing of the vocal fold tissue. A person's ability to produce voice with good quality largely depends on how well the injured tissue is restored. Therefore, understanding the process of wound healing is crucial.

Wound Healing Process

The goal of the wound healing process is to restore structure and function of the original tissue. It is a highly complex process in which numerous cells and extracellular constituents interact. Successful wound healing requires a highly regulated and well-orchestrated process. Failure to go through this process in a timely and orderly manner results in unsuccessful wound healing. The process of wound healing can be broken down into four phases: hemostasis, inflammation, proliferation, and remodeling (Diegelmann & Evans, 2004). A number of biological events occur in each phase and have distinct mechanisms but are not independent of each other, and there is considerable overlap from one phase to the next. How well one event is completed significantly influences the outcome of the following event. A brief description of the general wound healing process is given below.

Hemostasis Phase

Wound healing begins immediately after the injury. The first event in wound healing is hemostasis, a process that stops the bleeding. Hemostasis is achieved in three stages: vascular constriction, platelet plug formation, and coagulation (Sherwood, 2012). Upon injury, the blood vessels constrict to decrease blood loss. Platelets in the blood adhere to exposed collagen and other extracellular matrix (ECM) molecules of the blood vessel tissue and become activated. The activated platelets secrete mediators and adhesive proteins that help other platelets to further aggregate and adhere to the wound site in order to form a platelet plug (Li, Chen, & Kirsner, 2007). The blood contains proteins called coagulation factors, which become activated by the platelet aggregation and tissue factors (i.e., a membrane protein present in the vascular tissue) (Dahlback, 2000). These factors then undergo a process called the coagulation cascade, a series of complex biochemical reactions specialized for clot formation (Sherwood). The activated platelets and other constituents of the platelet plug, such as collagen, thrombin, and fibronectin, release cytokines and growth factors that are important for attracting white blood cells to the injury site (Broughton, Janis, & Attinge, 2006a).

Inflammatory Phase

The inflammatory phase follows the hemostasis phase. Inflammation is a normal and essential process of wound healing (Eming, Krieg, & Davidson, 2007; Koh & DiPietro, 2011). Timely resolution of inflammation is crucial for successful wound repair (Eming et al.). The inflammatory phase involves vascular and cellular components that interact and progress in parallel (Stadelmann, Digenis, & Tobin, 1998a). The blood vessels that became constricted during the hemostasis phase begin to dilate, and this dilation of the blood vessels increases the permeability of the blood vessel wall, allowing a variety of cells in the blood to leave the blood vessels to go to the injury site (Stadelmann et al., 1998a).

White blood cells (also called leukocytes or immune cells) are the main cellular players of this phase (Eming et al., 2007; Stadelmann et al., 1998a). Among different types of the white blood cells, polymorphonuclear neutrophils (PMNs) are the first ones that arrive to the injury site via the cytokine released from the hemostatic plug (Broughton et al.,

2006a; Stadelmann et al., 1998a; Digenis, & Tobin, 1998). PMNs begin clearing debridement of damaged tissue and infectious agents. Monocytes then arrive to the injury site and differentiate into macrophages as they exit from the blood vessels. Macrophages play many important roles in the inflammatory phase as they engulf and digest debris of cells and damaged tissues. Macrophages also serve as an antigen presenting cell upon digestion of a pathogen, and initiate an adaptive immune response via T-cells. Cytokines in the wound amplify the inflammatory response of the macrophage (Eming et al., 2007). Macrophages also synthesize various enzymes, cytokines, and growth factors (Broughton et al., 2006a). Together, these cytokines and growth factors help attract and activate fibroblasts, which are the cells that play important roles in the following proliferation phase.

Proliferation Phase

As the inflammation subsides, the proliferation phase begins. In this phase, several critical events for forming new tissue take place. These events include epithelialization, angiogenesis, granulation tissue formation, and collagen deposition (Broughton et al., 2006a). During epithelialization (the first event), a cytokine tumor necrosis factor alpha (TNF-α) secreted from active platelets and macrophages stimulates the epithelial cells on the wound edge to begin to proliferate and migrate. This activity restores the barrier function of the epithelium. Endothelial cells then begin angiogenesis, the second event, stimulated also by TNF-α, and vascular endothelial growth factor (VEGF), which is secreted from macrophages, platelets, and fibroblasts (Broughton, Janis, & Attinger, 2006b). The newly formed capillaries provide the nutrients required for formation of the granulation tissue that follows. Granulation tissue replaces the fibrin matrix formed during the hemostasis phase and serves as a new foundation for migration of the epithelial cells.

The fibroblasts are the main cellular player of the proliferation phase. As mentioned earlier, macrophages secrete TNF-α and platelet-derived growth factor (PDGF), which attract fibroblasts from surrounding tissue or bone marrow. These cytokine and growth factors also help fibroblasts proliferate (Broughton et al., 2006a; Gurtner, Werner, Barrandon, & Longaker, 2008). Matrix metalloproteinases (MMPs) that are secreted by macrophages, monocytes, and fibroblasts (Broughton et al., 2006b) degrade the tightly woven ECM and allow more fibroblasts to migrate into the wound site from the surrounding tissue and/or bone marrow (Singer & Clark, 1999). Macrophages also secrete transforming growth factor–β1 (TGF-β1), which stimulates or inhibits cellular proliferation depending on its concentration (Broughton et al., 2006a). TGF-β1 also stimulates fibroblasts to secrete various ECM constituents, such as collagen, glycosaminoglycans (GAGs), and proteoglycans (Sorrell & Caplan, 2009). Some of the fibroblasts differentiate into myofibroblasts, which are characterized by actin-containing microfilaments that give the cells the ability to contract and close the wound (Broughton et al., 2006b; Singer & Clark). This differentiation process is also driven by TGF-β1.

Remodeling/Maturation Phase

Remodeling is the last phase of wound healing. In this phase, restoration of the functional and structural integrity of newly formed tissue is completed (Li et al., 2007). Initially, the constituents in the provisional ECM are haphazardly organized. However, during remodeling, the haphazardly organized ECM is gradually replaced by a more organized and stronger collagenous matrix. This process is also affected by the chemical and mechanical environment of the wound. When enough collagen matrix is deposited, fibroblasts stop its synthesis and secretion (Singer & Clark, 1999) and any unnecessary endothelial cells, macrophages, and myofibroblasts undergo cell death (apoptosis) or leave the wound site (Gurtner et al., 2008). Degradation activity of MMPs is counterbalanced by tissue inhibitors of metalloproteases (TIMPs) (Broughton et al., 2006b). This balance must be well regulated for achieving successful wound healing (Baker & Leaper, 2003). The remodeling phase can last over 6 to 12 months, and constituents of the ECM are actively replaced and reorganized during that time to approximate the original tissue.

Factors That Influence Wound Healing

As described above, a number of biological events occur in each phase of wound healing, and each event has a distinct mechanism. These events are not independent of each other, and there is considerable overlap from one phase to the next. How well one event is completed significantly influences the outcome of the following event, and ultimately, the final outcome.

A number of other factors are also known to impede the wound healing process. These factors are divided into systemic and local categories. Systemic factors include age, smoking, alcohol consumption, obesity, stress (Kiecolt-Glaser, Marucha, Malarkey, Mercado, & Glaser, 2005), nutrition, presence of chronic metabolic disorders such as diabetes mellitus, genetic predisposition (Brown & Bayat, 2009), and use of systemic glucocorticoid steroids and nonsteroidal anti-inflammatory drugs (NSAIDs) (Stadelmann et al., 1998b; Guo & Dipietro, 2010). Local factors include excessive mechanical stress, hypoxia, infection, presence of foreign body, and venous insufficiency (Stadelmann et al., 1998b; Guo & Dipietro).

Scarring

Wound healing in postnatal life is a reparative rather than regenerative process. The resultant tissue is therefore only an approximation of lost tissue, which means that even a successful healing process results in some degree of scarring. Matured scar tissue is typically less vascular, consists of fewer cells (Greenhalgh, 1998), and has suboptimal mechanical properties compared with the original tissue (Broughton et al., 2006a). Unsuccessful tissue healing results in excessive scarring. Clinically, scar tissue becomes a problem when it fails to perform a required biological function.

Although inflammation is a necessary step for wound healing, prolonged inflammation leads to scarring. Chronic inflammation disturbs balance between proteolytic enzymes and their inhibitors that is crucial for ECM repair (Eming, Krieg, & Davidson, 2007). Excessive proliferation of granulation tissue, excessive deposition of fibrous proteins, inadequate degradation of excess ECM proteins, and excessive contraction of tissue are also some of the mechanisms that lead to scarring.

TGF-β has been extensively investigated due to its multifunctionality in the wound healing process and its role in scar formation. In the early phase of wound healing, TGF-β is secreted by the activated platelets as they degranulate and attract macrophages to the wound site (Martin, 1997; Barrientos, Stojadinovic, Golinko, Brem, & Tomic-Canic, 2008). Activated TGF-β1 stimulates fibroblast proliferation and collagen synthesis, therefore overabundance of TGF-β1 results in excessive deposition of collagen at the wound site, leading to scarring. TGF-β1 also prompts fibroblasts to differentiate into myofibroblasts

in the remodeling phase (Martin, 1997). The contractile property of myofibroblasts helps close the wound; however, untimely apoptosis of myofibroblasts will continue to exert mechanical loading on the ECM (Martin, 1997). Overabundance of TGF-β1 in the wound site perpetuates fibroblast-myofibroblast differentiation and causes persistent mechanical loading. Unloading of the mechanical force on the cells is important, as it cues apoptosis of myofibroblasts. Neutralization of TGF-β1 has been shown to reduce scarring (Martin, 1997). Anti-TGF-β therapy has shown promising results in animal models for scar reduction, and its effect is under investigation in clinical trial studies (Liu, Wu, & Gao, 2011).

Vocal Fold Wound Healing and Scar

The understanding of the vocal fold wound healing process and underlying biological mechanism of vocal fold pathologies has grown tremendously in the last 2 decades. Vocal fold wound healing studies have shown that vocal fold tissues follow a general progression of the wound healing process. The hemostasis phase lasts about 24 hours, inflammation phase continues for 4 to 7 days, and completion of re-epithelialization is seen approximately 7 days after the injury (Cho, Kim, Lee, Kim, & Park 2000; Thibeault & Gray, 2005).

A resulting vocal fold scar is not uncommon and remains as a major challenge in the care of voice disorders. Research studies have shown that scarred vocal fold tissue is stiffer than uninjured vocal fold tissue and thus not able to vibrate like healthy, unscarred tissue (Hertegard, Dahlqvist, & Goodyer, 2006; Thibeault, Gray, Bless, Chan & Ford, 2002). Scarred vocal fold tissue is characterized by disorganized collagen scaffolding and altered levels of ECM constituents. Significantly less collagen, an increase in procollagen, and a decrease in elastin compared with normal vocal fold lamina propria have been reported (Thibeault et al., 2002). Currently, there is no effective treatment for established scar tissue (Hirano, 2005; Wolfram, Tzankov, Pulzl, & Piza-Katzer, 2009). Researchers are studying the potential of novel treatment approaches, such as tissue engineering, growth factor therapy, and stem cell therapy, for preventing excessive scar formation (Gaston, Quinchia Rios, Bartlett, Berchtold, & Thibeault, 2012; Hong et al., 2011; Kutty & Webb, 2009; Long, 2010; Ohno et al., 2011, 2012; Suehiro et al., 2010; Svensson et al., 2011)

Voice Therapy and Wound Healing

The role of voice therapy in promoting vocal fold wound healing is poorly understood. Clinical experience and limited literature on voice rest suggest that postsurgical voice rest (as opposed to uncontrolled phonation) appears to facilitate vocal fold wound healing better in the early stages of healing (Ishikawa & Thibeault, 2010). Currently, voice therapy has a role in reducing excessive mechanical stress to the vocal fold tissue to prevent further injury. The impact of applying mechanical stress during the wound healing process has been extensively studied in other types of connective tissue, such as knee ligament. The orthopedic literature indicates that mobilization of tissue is more favorable than immobilization; however, the effect on healing depends on dose, magnitude, and type of stress (Ishikawa & Thibeault, 2010). Although both ligaments and lamina propria are connective tissue, whether the findings in the orthopedic literature can be directly applied to vocal fold wound healing is entirely unknown. A recent study suggested that voice exercises may have a positive impact on attenuating acute inflammation (Verdolini Abbott et al., 2012), but there is still much to be discovered. The facilitative role of voice exercises in vocal fold wound healing is an intriguing question for future studies.

References

Baker, E. A., & Leaper, D. J. (2003). Profiles of matrix metalloproteinases and their tissue inhibitors in intraperitoneal drainage fluid: Relationship to wound healing. *Wound Repair and Regeneration, 11*, 268–274.

Barrientos, S., Stojadinovic, O., Golinko, M. S., Brem, H., & Tomic-Canic, M. (2008). Growth factors and cytokines in wound healing. *Wound Repair and Regeneration, 16*, 585–601.

Broughton, G., 2nd, Janis, J. E., & Attinger, C. E. (2006a). Wound healing: An overview. *Plastic and Reconstructive Surgery, 117*(7 Suppl), 1eS–32eS.

Broughton, G., 2nd, Janis, J. E., & Attinger, C. E. (2006b). The basic science of wound healing. *Plastic and Reconstructive Surgery, 117*, 12S–34S.

Brown, J. J., & Bayat, A. (2009). Genetic susceptibility to raised dermal scarring. *British Journal of Dermatology, 161*, 8–18.

Cho, S. H., Kim, H. T., Lee, I. J., Kim, M. S., & Park, H. J. (2000). Influence of phonation on basement membrane zone recovery after phonomicrosurgery: A canine model. *The Annals of Otology, Rhinology, and Laryngology, 109*, 658–666.

Dahlback, B. (2000). Blood coagulation. *Lancet, 355*, 1627–1632.

Diegelmann, R. F., & Evans, M. C. (2004). Wound healing: An overview of acute, fibrotic and delayed healing. *Frontiers in Bioscience, 9*, 283–289.

Eming, S. A., Krieg, T., & Davidson, J. M. (2007). Inflammation in wound repair: Molecular and cellular mechanisms. *Journal of Investigative Dermatology, 127*, 514–552

Gaston, J., Quinchia Rios, B., Bartlett, R., Berchtold, C., & Thibeault, S. L. (2012). The response of vocal fold fibroblasts and mesenchymal stromal cells to vibration. *PLoS*

ONE, *7*(2), e30965. doi:10.1371/journal .pone.0030965

Greenhalgh, D. G. (1998). The role of apoptosis in wound healing. *International Journal of Biochemistry and Cell Biology, 30,* 1019–1030.

Gurtner, G. C., Werner, S., Barrandon, Y., & Longaker, M. T. (2008). Wound repair and regeneration. *Nature, 453,* 314–321.

Guo, S., & Dipietro, L. A. (2010). Factors affecting wound healing. *Journal of Dental Research, 89,* 219–229.

Hertegard, S., Dahlqvist, A., & Goodyer, E. (2006). Viscoelastic measurements after vocal fold scarring in rabbits—short-term results after hyaluronan injection. *Acta Otolaryngologica, 126,* 758–763.

Hirano, S. (2005). Current treatment of vocal fold scarring. *Current Opinion in Otolaryngology and Head and Neck Surgery, 13,* 143–147.

Hong, S. J., Lee, S. H., Jin, S. M., Kwon, S. Y., Jung, K. Y., Kim, M. K., . . . Lee, K. W. (2011). Vocal fold wound healing after injection of human adipose-derived stem cells in a rabbit model. *Acta Otolaryngologica, 131,* 1198–1204.

Ishikawa, K., & Thibeault, S. (2010). Voice rest versus exercise: A review of the literature. *Journal of Voice, 24,* 379–387.

Kiecolt-Glaser, J. K., Marucha, P. T., Malarkey, W. B., Mercado, A. M., & Glaser, R. (1995). Slowing of wound healing by psychological stress. *Lancet, 346,* 1194–1196.

Koh, T. J., & DiPietro, L. A. (2011). Inflammation and wound healing: The role of the macrophage. *Expert Reviews in Molecular Medicine, 13,* e23.

Kutty, J. K., & Webb, K. (2009). Tissue engineering therapies for the vocal fold lamina propria. *Tissue Engineering Part B: Reviews, 15,* 249–262.

Li, J., Chen, J., & Kirsner, R. (2007). Pathophysiology of acute wound healing. *Clinics in Dermatology, 25,* 9–18.

Liu, W., Wu, X., & Gao, Z. (2011). New potential antiscarring approaches. *Wound Repair and Regeneration, 19*(Suppl. 1), s22–s31.

Long, J. L. (2010). Tissue engineering for treatment of vocal fold scar. *Current Opinion in Otolaryngology & Head and Neck Surgery, 18,* 521–525.

Martin, P. (1997). Wound healing-aiming for perfect skin regeneration. *Science, 276,* 75–81.

Ohno, S., Hirano, S., Kanemaru, S., Kitani, Y., Kojima, T., Ishikawa, S., . . . Ito, J. (2012). Transforming growth factor beta-3 for the prevention of vocal fold scarring. *Laryngoscope, 122,* 583–589.

Ohno, S., Hirano, S., Kanemaru, S., Kitani, Y., Kojima, T., Tateya, I., . . . Ito, J. (2011). Implantation of an atelocollagen sponge with autologous bone marrow-derived mesenchymal stromal cells for treatment of vocal fold scarring in a canine model. *Annals of Otology, Rhinology, and Laryngology, 120,* 401–408.

Sherwood, L. (2012). *Human physiology: From cells to systems.* Stamford, CT: Cengage Learning.

Singer, A. J., & Clark, R. A. (1999). Cutaneous wound healing. *New England Journal of Medicine, 341,* 738–746.

Sorrell, J. M., & Caplan, A. (2009). Fibroblasts— a diverse population at the center of it all. *International Review of Cell and Molecular Biology, 276,* 161–214.

Stadelmann, W. K., Digenis, A. G., Tobin, G. R. (1998a). Physiology and healing dynamics of chronic cutaneous wounds. *American Journal of Surgery, 176,* 26S–38S.

Stadelmann, W. K., Digenis, A. G., & Tobin, G. R. (1998b). Impediments to wound healing. *American Journal of Surgery, 176,* 39S–47S.

Suehiro, A., Hirano, S., Kishimoto, Y., Tateya, I., Rousseau, B., & Ito, J. (2010). Effects of basic fibroblast growth factor on rat vocal fold fibroblasts. *Annals of Otology, Rhinology, and Laryngology, 119,* 690–696.

Svensson, B., Nagubothu, S. R., Cedervall, J., Chan, R. W., Le Blanc, K., Kimura, M., . . . Hertegard, S. (2011). Injection of human mesenchymal stem cells improves healing of vocal folds after scar excision—a xenograft analysis. *Laryngoscope, 121,* 2185–2190.

Thibeault, S. L., & Gray, S. D. (2005). Vocal fold injury and repair. In R. T. Sataloff (Ed.), *Voice Science* (pp. 105–113). San Diego, CA: Plural Publishing.

Thibeault, S. L., Gray, S. D., Bless, D. M., Chan, R. W., & Ford, C. N. (2002). Histologic and rheologic characterization of vocal fold scarring. *Journal of Voice, 16*, 96–104.

Verdolini Abbott, K., Li, N. Y., Branski, R. C., Rosen, C. A., Grillo, E., Steinhauer, K., & Hebda, P. A. (2012). Vocal exercise may attenuate acute vocal fold inflammation. *Journal of Voice, 26*, 814.e1–814.e13.

Wolfram, D., Tzankov, A., Pulzl, P., & Piza-Katzer, H. (2009). Hypertrophic scars and keloids—a review of their pathophysiology, risk factors, and therapeutic management. *Dermatologic Surgery, 35*, 171–181.

Index

Note: Color Plates are numbered consecutively with the Color Plate page numbers preceded by CP. Page numbers in **bold** reference non-text material.